Working with AIDS Bereavement

A Comprehensive Approach for Mental Health Providers

Peter B Goldblum PhD MPH
Sarah Erickson PhD

UCSF AIDS Health Project Monograph Series Number Three
Published by the AIDS Health Project, University of California San Francisco
Monograph Series Editors: James W. Dilley, MD and Robert Marks

First Printing, October 1999. Printed in the United States of America.

LIBRARY OF CONGRESS CATALOGING-IN-PUBLICATION DATA

Goldblum, Peter.

Working with AIDS Bereavement : a comprehensive approach for mental health providers / Peter B. Goldblum, Sarah Erickson.

p. cm. -- (UCSF AIDS Health Project monograph series; no. 3)

Includes bibliographical references and index.

ISBN 1-879168-03-0 (pbk.)

1. Bereavement--Psychological aspects. 2. Grief. 3. Death--Psychological aspects. 4. Loss (Psychology) 5. AIDS (Disease)--Psychological aspects. I. Erickson, Sarah, 1964– II. Title. III. Series.

BF575.G7 G684 1999

155.9'37--dc21 99-047163

UCSF AIDS HEALTH PROJECT, Box 0884, San Francisco, CA 94143-0884.

James W. Dilley, MD, Executive Director. Joanna Rinaldi, Deputy Director. Robert Marks, Director of Publications and Training, Editor. Shauna O'Donnell, John Tighe, Editorial assistance. Saul Rosenfield, Book design. Saul Rosenfield, Cover design. Sayre Van Young, Indexing. Andrew Tavoni, Production. Kathy Barr, Shauna O'Donnell, Proofreading. Carrel Crawford, Distribution. Carrel Crawford, Shauna O'Donnell, Administrative support. Alex Chase, Pegoh Pajouhi, Cybele Tom, Research and production support.

The AIDS Health Project is an affiliated unit of the Langley Porter Psychiatric Institute, School of Medicine, University of California San Francisco.

DONATIONS AND GRANTS. Typefaces donated by Adobe Systems, Mountain View, California. We thank Adobe for its generosity.

Funding for this book from the California Department of Mental Health: Gray Davis, Governor; Grantland Johnson, Secretary, Health and Welfare Agency; Stephen W. Mayberg, PHD, Director of Mental Health, California Department of Mental Health.

PERMISSIONS. The following have generously granted permission for use of copyrighted work: Baywood Publishing Co., Inc. for an extended quotation from *Heavenly Hurts: Surviving AIDs Related Deaths and Losses* by Sandra Jacoby Klein, copyright 1998 by Sandra Jacoby Klein. Lippincott Williams & Wilkins for use of a chart on the diagnostic criteria for pathological grief that ran in the journal *Psychosomatic Medicine*, copyright 1993. The NAMES Project Foundation for the three "true stories," previously printed in *On Display*, the project's newsletter, copyright 1999 by William Aull, 1998 by Lucille C. Sansevero, 1998 by Rosetta Dubois-Gadsen. The artist Domenic Ali, who graciously modified a detail of his print *Witness* (copyright 1996 by Domenic Ali) for use on the cover.

Contents

UCSF AIDS Health Project Monographs

THE UCSF AIDS HEALTH PROJECT, affiliated with the Langley Porter Psychiatric Institute of the University of California San Francisco's world-renowned medical school, is a leader in developing clinical services and professional education to meet the mental health needs of people affected by HIV disease. Since 1984, AHP has been nationally recognized for pioneering programs in a variety of areas, including HIV-related counseling and support, antibody testing and counseling, and HIV-related substance abuse services.

The UCSF AIDS Health Project Monograph Series, underwritten by the California Department of Mental Health, offers clear, concise, and practical information on HIV-related topics of particular concern to mental health providers. The first book in the series was *AIDS and the Impact of Cognitive Impairment: A Treatment Guide for Mental Health Providers* ($7.95). The second book in the series was *The Alcohol and Drug Wildcard: Substance Use and Psychiatric Problems in People with HIV* ($9.95).

UCSF AIDS Health Project Publications

AHP publishes a range of other publications for mental health and health care providers. AHP published what has become a standard in HIV counseling primers, *Face to Face: A Guide to AIDS Counseling* ($16.95). In late 1998, AHP joined with Jossey-Bass Publishers, Inc. to publish a successor to this volume: *The UCSF AIDS Health Project Guide to Counseling: Perspectives on Psychotherapy, Prevention, and Therapeutic Practice* ($27.95; direct price).

In addition, AHP has published other books for mental health providers, including: *Risk and Recovery: AIDS, HIV, and Alcohol* ($16.95) and *AIDS Law for Mental Health Professionals: A Guide to Judicious Practice* ($19.95).

Finally, AHP publishes several newsletters, including *FOCUS: A Guide to AIDS Research and Counseling*, one of the longest-running HIV-related newsletters in the country. *FOCUS*, which has an international reputation, reviews the counseling aspects of HIV disease and is an indispensible reference for counselors, health care providers, and scholars ($36.00 for an individual subscription; $90.00 for an institutional subscription: international rates available). AHP also publishes the *FOCUS Supplement on Antibody Test Counseling* and *HIV Counselor PERSPECTIVES*, both of which are newsletters for antibody test counselors.

For more information or to order AHP publications, please write UCSF AIDS Health Project, Box 0884, San Francisco, CA 94143-0884; call 415-502-7270; fax 415-476-7996; or visit our web site: www.ucsf-ahp.org.

Contributors

Peter B. Goldblum, PhD, MPH is the Director of the Stanford AIDS Caregiving and Bereavement Study and a clinical psychologist in private practice in San Francisco. He was a founder and Deputy Director of the UCSF AIDS Health Project and is an Associate Professor of Psychology at the Pacific Graduate School of Psychology in Palo Alto, Calif.

Sarah Erickson, PhD is an Assistant Professor in Clinical Psychology at the University of New Mexico, Albuquerque. She completed her doctorate and postdoctoral fellowship at Stanford University, where she co-directed the Stanford Caregiving and Bereavement Study. She also worked at the UCSF Center for AIDS Prevention Studies, gaining additional insight into the lives and challenges of people with AIDS.

Acknowledgments

Putting a monograph like this together requires the efforts of many people. The authors and the editors extend their appreciation to UCSF AIDS Health Project staff and volunteers who contributed to the process. (See the copyright page for a list of these individuals.) In addition, the authors wish to especially acknowledge the following people.

This monograph has been a long time in the making. Originally conceived as an expansion of a previously written book chapter entitled "The Clinical Management of Bereavement" for The UCSF AIDS Health Project Guide to Counseling *(Jossey-Bass, 1998), the project evolved into an articulation of a new model for understanding bereavement. This model relies on the work of several contemporary bereavement theorists and researchers: we are particularly indebted to Susan Folkman, Mardi Horowitz, and Camille Wortman and their colleagues for guiding the way for empirically grounded clinical approaches for assisting mourners.*

This monograph could not have been produced without the tireless efforts of its two editors: Rob Marks and Jim Dilley. First of all, they allowed us the opportunity to write the monograph. But more importantly, they shepherded us through the process, challenging us to articulate our thinking, and reviewing version after version for inconsistencies and inaccuracies. We have benefited from their patience, insight, and humanity, all an integral part of the underlying fabric of this work.

Michael Carr's contributions to the monograph were also essential. As the Director of Art and Archive for the AIDS Memorial Quilt and editor of its newsletter On Display, *he was instru-*

mental in procuring and preparing the three True Stories included in the monograph. As Peter's life partner, his love, support, and encouragement – not to mention the wonderful meals he prepared – were of the greatest comfort. Scott Webster, Sarah's partner, provided support, encouragement, patience, and good camaraderie throughout the process.

We also want to acknowledge the tremendous contributions of Susan Nolen-Hoeksema, who afforded us the initial opportunity to conduct the Stanford AIDS Caregiving and Bereavement Study, and provided conceptual guidance and inspiration throughout her stay at Stanford. Other Stanford colleagues helped collect and analyze the study data. Robert Witlox, joining us from Amsterdam, provided fresh perspective and much hard work.

Many people helped prepare the manuscript for the monograph. Stephen Shuchter provided sage advice regarding the use of pharmacological interventions and reviewed the final manuscript. Sally Reid, Louise Gaston, and Barbara Davis reviewed versions of the manuscript and provided theoretical and clinical insights. Staff members of the UCSF AIDS Health Project diligently reviewed various versions and provided excellent editorial work.

Finally, we would like to express our profound appreciation to the AIDS mourners who participated in the Stanford study for sharing their lives and insights with us. Many participants stated their involvement in the study was a form of memorial to their loved ones lost to AIDS. We are grateful to them for allowing us to be a part of their mourning process.

– Peter Goldblum, PhD, MPH

– Sarah Erickson, PhD

Prologue: A Personal and Professional Journey

I remember that first time in the early 1980s when I walked into a hospital room as a psychologist to counsel a dying patient with what was then termed "Gay Cancer." When my colleague, Patrick McGraw, called with the referral, he spoke in a sad tone with a touch of irony in it, "I've done all I can do for him medically. This is the time I usually ask the chaplain to go in, but neither Ron nor his lover, Sidney, feel comfortable with a priest or rabbi, so I thought a psychotherapist would do. Anyway, I figured you'd know what to do."

At first I was flattered, then bewildered; nothing in my psychological training prepared me to make such a visit. As I walked up the steps to the hospital, the words "compassionate care" kept coming to my mind.

When I entered the room, I found a gravely ill man in the hospital bed, his partner standing next to him holding his hand. They were expecting my visit and welcomed me cautiously. Trained by frequent visits from medical consultants, the couple fell into telling me

Ron's medical history. I was glad they did, because it gave me time to think about what I had to offer these men. When a nurse came in to do a brief medical procedure for Ron, I got another reprieve.

In the hallway with Ron's partner, Sidney, I asked him how he was doing. Obviously exhausted, he bravely reassured me that he was holding up. I then asked him if there was anything that he wanted to say – or wanted to hear – from Ron that wasn't being said. At first Sidney seemed surprised by the question, but then relief spread over his face. "Well, yes there is," he said. "Ron and I have been together for fourteen years. We have a beautiful home together and raise prize show dogs. We get along wonderfully. Neither of us is what you would call 'mushy'; we haven't had sex in years, and that's fine with both of us. I know that he loves me and would do anything for me, but neither of us has said that to the other for a long time. I would like to hear him say he loves me and I want to tell him how much I love him, but I feel embarrassed." I asked if he would like me to help them have that discussion, and he said he would.

Relieved to have a purpose, I returned to the room with Sidney. I told Ron that the reason for my visit was to help him and Sidney say those things they wanted to say to each other before they had to say good-bye. Since no one really understood the disease that he had, no one could really predict the future. Ron broke in at that point and said, " I know that I'm dying. I need to start saying my good-byes."

Ron started out in a weak and frail voice. "Sidney, I know that I don't say this as often as I should, but I really want you to know how much I love you and that my only regret about dying is leaving you." All three of us began to cry, as Sidney proclaimed his unending love. Shortly, I excused myself, gave them my card, and said I would check in over the next few days.

Two days later Sidney called to tell me that Ron had died peacefully. He thanked me and told me that the last two days were the closest of their lives. Again, with a quiver in my voice, I encouraged him to check in with me whenever he needed. I did not hear from Sidney for several months; then he called and came by my office for one session. He wept as he described the last days of Ron's life. When I asked Sidney how he was doing now, he said that he was progressing well – busy with the house, garden, and dogs. As he was leaving he said, "I just want you to know what a comfort it is for me knowing and having heard from Ron that he loved me. Thank you."

Witnessing Bereavement

I learned many things that day with Ron and Sidney. First, bereavement work begins long before a person experiences a death. Getting respectful, compassionate care from medical providers, having your relationship honored by others, and knowing that you have done a good job caring for a loved one: all of these go a long way toward facilitating the mourning process. Second, at the core of what we as mental health professionals do is compassion. Our ability to be present with our clients and to listen with an open heart will usually guide us to do the right thing. Finally, compassion and knowledge augment and potentiate each other: knowing what we are doing – what is expected of us – allows us to focus more compassionately on our clients' needs rather than our own insecurities.

Over the years since I met Ron and Sidney, I have watched as AIDS has compelled so many of us to face our mortality: many have died, many more live on infected, and all of us know more profoundly than we did about the temporary nature of life. For those of us who have weathered the losses of the epidemic, the threat of becoming overwhelmed and demoralized is a real danger. As therapists working on the front lines, we run the real risk of falling into what has been termed "empathy fatigue." I know, for I have been there.

I particularly remember the trying times during the final days of my partner Kenny's life. With the help of a wonderful group of colleagues, I found the courage to discuss my situation openly with each of my clients. To my surprise, I received nothing but the kindest support from each, and together, we were able to define a suitable course of action: some went temporarily or permanently to other therapists; others took a break from therapy and returned later. I have never viewed my clients in exactly the same way again.

After Kenny's death, I took a two-year break from doing psychotherapy. In 1989, I became interested in doing research on AIDS bereavement. A friend of mine who worked for the AIDS hospice program at the San Francisco Visiting Nurse Association referred me to Susan Nolen-Hoeksema, a teacher and researcher at Stanford, who was the principle investigator of a large bereavement study funded by the National Institutes of Health. The suggestion was timely, given Susan's interest in expanding her research to include the AIDS bereaved. Soon, she invited me to join her bereavement research group and work with her then-graduate student Sarah Erickson to develop the AIDS Caregiving and Bereavement Study.

My experience at Stanford opened my eyes to the complexity of the study of bereavement in general. I came to realize the gulf between clinical lore and empirical evidence. Further, I was exposed to two apparently opposing theoretical and research traditions: the more empirically driven stress and coping model and the more theoretically driven psychodynamic model. At times I felt like a fish out of water; surrounded by highly skilled, technologically sophisticated researchers, I often heard disparaging remarks about "soft thinking" clinicians. At other times, I felt that these "egg heads" totally missed the point and were more interested in statistical significance than real life significance. Fortunately, I had an ally in Sarah, who is one of those amazing people who is equally comfortable in both worlds. We spent many hours – which usually included enjoying a nice meal and some gossip – trying to reconcile these two perspectives. I like to think that we have grappled with these issues in a way that is "tough minded and kind hearted" (a term used to describe the late Congresswoman Barbara Jordan).

Since returning to psychotherapy, I have been privileged to work with many gay men grieving AIDS losses. Some have lost romantic relationships, others grieve the loss of deep friendships. I have come to think of all of these stories as love stories. Each contradicts the homophobic belief that gay men do not form deep emotional attachments. Each has taught me the art of loving: the ways relationships start, how attachments form, and how affection can deepen over time. As with any love story, most include conflicts, some that resolve, some that remain.

True Story One: William and David

This monograph includes three "true stories" to more genuinely reflect the experience of AIDS mourners. The first, below, is an excerpt from a letter sent by William Aull, a nurse at the Rainbow Home in Pennsylvania, to the editor of *On Display*, the newsletter of the AIDS Memorial Quilt. William's is a common but rarely told story. As health care providers, we often develop deep emotions for our patients; occasionally an especially deep relationship forms.

> *I, like many other professional caregivers, have had many friends who have died from AIDS – too many to count. I did not know David prior to his admission to Rainbow Home, but I grew to know him very quickly and I want to share my experiences as his caregiver and*

friend. David came to us from a nursing home in another state. . . . He was very angry and I could understand why he felt this way.

David was one of the lucky ones – he had tremendous family support. His mom and several of his aunts were nurses and would spend as much time with him as possible. . . . I finally had someone with whom I could discuss opera. I prefer Leontyne Price – David had other favorites. . . . He also liked Barbra Streisand and Madonna, so we'd listen to these tapes together while I was performing care.

David longed to get out into the world and see things. He simply wasn't ready to sit and watch TV all day. We had a lot of work ahead of us. He had minimal use of his legs, but was determined to walk again. We hoped the "cocktails" his new doctor prescribed might be the key to his dream of walking. We worked long and hard on range-of-motion activities. Our duo wasn't about to give up the ship! David's legs eventually strengthened to the point where he could walk for short periods of time. Our most joyous day was the day he and I went to Sunday Mass and he was able to get into and out of the car on his own. It was a miracle! . . .

A week after David and I attended Mass – just one week after his great triumph of walking – he took a sudden and unexpected turn for the worse. I was blessed that my co-worker understood how important David had become to me and she set me free to help David through the dying process. Hour by hour his condition worsened and he kept asking me not to leave him. At 2:18 p.m. on January 5, with his head on my right shoulder and his family by his side, listening to Madonna, David went to God. He died with dignity and respect, pain-free, surrounded by those who loved him.

My grief actually started the morning David started to deteriorate. When David died on my shoulder I knew the end had come, but I couldn't move. I needed that bond to send him to God. I remember laying my head on his chest and sobbing. Then I went about my duties notifying the rest of the staff, calling the priest and gathering his belongings. It was shift change and the woman who replaced me graciously gave me permission to prepare the body for the funeral director. We are family at Rainbow Home and this is one of the ways we help each other cope.

I had to leave before the funeral director arrived because the pain was so great. Besides, I had promised David I would do something if "that time came." I went to a local bar and all of us there drank a toast to David. It's months later and I'm still healing. I know it will take a long time. He was very special to me.

As frequently as these special relationships happen, little is written or taught about how to manage them. As wonderful as these relationships are, they can also be confusing given their mixed professional and personal nature. Because these relationships are not widely discussed, they sometimes make other co-workers a bit uneasy and families sometimes feel displaced by their intensity.

On the other hand, too often family and friends of the patient are unaware of the special nature of these relationships and professional caregivers are left out of final ceremonies, their role and their affection left unacknowledged. Fortunately, both William and David had solid support and validation for their friendship. David's family allowed William to join them before, during, and after David's death, including helping to make David's Quilt panel. William also received support from his colleagues, which will hopefully continue throughout his mourning process.

I am grateful to William for so candidly sharing his intimate story. Only as we openly tell stories of the deep bonds that we form with our clients can we begin to understand how to manage and mourn them. Yes, AIDS is both a nemesis and a teacher. The lessons learned are hard ones, and the losses are great. Each of us who confronts the disease and its losses must find his or her own strength to face its burdens and to find meaning within the struggle.

In the model we present in this monograph, we struggle to combine insights derived from the latest empirical and theoretical work with direct observations taken from our personal experiences and those of our clients. We have worked hard to soften the academic tone without losing too much in the way of precision. We have tried to provide a useful clinical model for the assessment and treatment of AIDS bereavement distress, while acknowledging that there still exist many unanswered questions. We have offered our own synthesis of a large and often contradictory literature on the subject. However, we have noted those areas where there continues to be disagreement or inconsistencies in the literature with the hope that the interested reader will hold these conclusions as tentative and will continue to follow future developments in the field.

– Peter Goldblum, PhD, MPH

Introduction: Overview and Definitions

AIDS mourners, and those who seek to assist them, face an ever-changing landscape of cultural and individual meanings related to the nature and social implications of HIV disease and the losses associated with the epidemic. These meanings profoundly affect an individual's response to loss and the success with which he or she resolves grief. The process of finding meaning in AIDS grief is facilitated by a well-grounded, comprehensive view of AIDS bereavement, a perspective that takes into account the historical and cultural contexts of AIDS bereavement and the psychological processes affecting AIDS mourning and grief. This monograph proposes such a perspective: the Integrative Model of AIDS Bereavement.

Contents

Chapter One lays the groundwork by discussing the historical, cultural, philosophical, and psychological contexts of mourning and specifically AIDS bereavement. Chapters Two and Three synthesize this material, borrowing from this library of theory the elements that comprise the Integrative Model, which will aid providers to assess and treat clients who need help navigating their mourning process.

The Integrative Model is based on empirical research, theory, and clinical observation related to both AIDS and general bereavement. This model is designed to help clinicians evaluate the type and level of bereavement distress experienced by an AIDS mourner, distinguish between uncomplicated and complicated grief, and determine whether a psychiatric disorder co-exists with grief. As part of this assessment, the monograph presents a procedure for evaluating risk factors for AIDS bereavement distress. This procedure is grounded in the latest findings in the AIDS and general bereavement literature.

The monograph then describes a range of bereavement activities and interventions and a method for matching AIDS mourners with appropriate bereavement activities on the basis of type and level of bereavement distress. Finally, the monograph proposes a psychotherapeutic approach – Integrative AIDS Bereavement Therapy – that combines aspects of both psychodynamic and cognitive behavioral therapy and is enhanced by recent developments specifically designed to assist AIDS mourners in preventing complicated grief.

Terminology

In a volume that seeks to synthesize the broad bereavement literature, the dilemma of selecting appropriate terminology is unavoidable. Even as the field explodes with new and sophisticated research on both bereavement in general and AIDS bereavement, there continues to be a lack of agreement regarding even basic terms. For example, *bereavement*, *grief*, and *mourning* are often used interchangeably. Further, there continues to be confusion regarding the proper term for grief or mourning that has gone awry, sometimes referred to as *pathological grief*, *pathological mourning*, or *complicated grief*.

In this monograph, basic terms of bereavement, grief, and mourning conform to definitions suggested by Margaret and Wolfgang Stroebe and Robert Hansson in *The Handbook of Bereavement*.[1] According to this convention, *bereavement* is the objective situation of having lost someone significant; *grief* is the emotional response to one's loss; and *mourning* denotes the actions and manner of expressing grief, which often reflect the mourning practices of one's culture.

Several terms have been specifically defined for this monograph. *Bereavement distress* encompasses both uncomplicated and complicated grief, and has been divided into four levels: uncomplicated grief, uncomplicated grief with risk factors, complicated grief without clinical disorder, and complicated grief with clinical disorder. *Uncomplicated grief* is defined as the adequate management of the grief process in which the mourner successfully moves through the phases and tasks of mourning consistent with his or her own values and cultural norms. *Complicated grief*, on the other hand, includes an atypical intensity or duration of grief symptoms that leads to a level of functional impairment in critical areas of work and relationships. Again, it is important to emphasize that this approach presumes that bereavement – even when characterized by uncomplicated grief and "the adequate management of the grief process" – causes distress.

For several reasons, the monograph uses the term *integrative* to describe both the overall model of bereavement and the process of bereavement therapy. First, both the model and therapy are multidisciplinary in approach. Observations from anthropology, sociology, and philosophy are joined with psychological views of mourning and grief to broaden and strengthen the perspective. Second, the monograph makes great efforts to synthesize and integrate insights garnered from both empirical research and clinical practice into a coherent whole. Finally, efforts to integrate findings from both psychodynamic and cognitive approaches appear in all aspects of the model: the underlying view of grief and mourning, the differential diagnosis of levels of bereavement distress, the selection of appropriate bereavement activities and interventions, and the application of these interventions.

Throughout the monograph, case materials illustrate theoretical and clinical principles. While based on actual clinical observations – by the monograph authors or sources found in the literature – most of these scenarios are amalgamations of several real-life examples, completely hypothetical cases, or actual examples that have been significantly altered to protect the confidentiality of clients. Furthermore, a noticeable bias toward case material with gay white men and their families reflects the clinical experience of the authors and the predominance of research and clinical writing in the field. To provide a more authentic picture of AIDS mourners, the monograph includes excerpts from three letters to the editor of *On*

Display, the newsletter of the AIDS Memorial Quilt. These "true stories" provide additional insights from actual individuals and families coping with the loss of a loved one to AIDS. The names in these cases are real and the letters are used with the permission of the authors.

Conclusion

Finally, as in so many other arenas of physical and psychosomatic medicine, the findings from research on and practice in AIDS bereavement has much to teach the broader field of bereavement support. Ideally, the model presented in this monograph will encourage other bereavement writers to combine historical, social, cultural, philosophical, and psychological perspectives into community and clinical approaches to assist other mourners. In the meantime, application of the principles presented here should serve clinicians well in their work with all mourners. If so – in some small way – this model will serve as a tribute to those who have died of AIDS and those who continue to work to help people with HIV and their loved ones.

1

The Meaning of AIDS Bereavement

MOURNING a loved one who has died from HIV disease presents both universal and unique challenges. To the extent that any of us allow ourselves to develop strong emotional attachments, we open ourselves to the experience of grief when these ties are severed. On the other hand, AIDS-related bereavement cannot be understood apart from the social, cultural, and symbolic context of HIV disease. The complexity, scope, focus, and process of the HIV epidemic are unique, coloring the burden of those who mourn its losses. To understand AIDS bereavement, therefore, it is important to understand both its commonality with general bereavement and its singularity.

It is useful to examine several overlapping areas of influence in order to recognize the most effective clinical approach to AIDS bereavement. Each of these areas plays a role in determining the context in which a person experiences a particular loss and the grief that follows; and each has been incorporated into the Integrative Model of AIDS Bereavement. Clinicians applying the model need to appreciate these influences upon the mourner and to be able to inquire specifically about an individual's experience along these lines. This chapter offers an overview of each of these areas as an introduction to the more practical application of assessment and treatment suggested in Chapters Two and Three. These four areas of influence are:

- The history of the epidemic;
- The cultural context of mourning;
- The philosophical perspective on life and death;
- The psychology of grief.

In reviewing these influences, this chapter considers, in particular, the U.S. experience with the epidemic. It is important to note that in many ways this experience is similar to that of other industrialized nations in Europe, but it is dramatically different from the experience in Africa, South America, and many parts of Asia.

The History of the Epidemic

AIDS has become a powerful symbol throughout the world, one that is capable of eliciting a variety of responses, including fear, hostility, hope and compassion. As a participant in an early HIV support group said, "In people's minds AIDS equals sex and death. This frightens them. Thus I frighten them."[2] On the other hand, anthropologist Mary Catherine Bateson writing in 1988 commented that, "AIDS moves along the fault lines of our society and becomes a metaphor for understanding that society. The AIDS epidemic, as it moves around the planet, is posing new questions about justice and teaching us new ways of thinking about human learning and human suffering."[3]

The history of the epidemic has been a history of both compassion and hostility. As cultures, communities, and individuals struggle to define appropriate reactions to HIV disease, they must reconcile contradictory cultural meanings regarding the disease, those infected, and the people who love and care for seropositive people and mourn their losses.

The Epidemic Unfolds

Initially, news and concern about HIV disease – before it was even called that – was fairly limited and centered mainly within the communities of urban gay men and people with hemophilia. The general public perceived little threat and the result was that government offered little support for publicly funded research. Eric Rofes, in *Reviving the Tribe,* described a dinner party in the early days of the epidemic: "Glazed-over eyes flashed about the room, each of us pondering who among us would be walking the earth in ten years. Serious discussion ensued about whether the gay male population was doomed for extinction."[4]

As the numbers of people with AIDS continued to grow and evidence suggested that the disease was contagious, public health providers focused more intensive attention on the condition. Over the next couple of years, researchers isolated and developed the HIV antibody test. Gradually, clinicians reported more cases of HIV disease among other populations, in North America and Europe, particularly among injection drug users and their sexual partners and among people of color. At the same time, awareness grew that HIV disease was a worldwide phenomenon spread heterosexually and rapidly in the non-industrialized world.[5]

On October 2, 1985, actor Rock Hudson died of AIDS. HIV disease became the topic of headlines throughout the world and a catalyst for heated debate regarding societal values related to privacy, individual freedom, and the need for social control. On the positive side, now that the disease had a face, many people outside those communities hardest hit began to approach the epidemic and those infected with less fear and more compassion.

By 1988, the rate of new infections was rising at an alarming rate. In the United States, 10,000 people had been diagnosed with HIV disease between 1981 and 1985. By 1988, 35,000 people were diagnosed and 20,000 people died. There was still no cure in sight. Eric Rofes described this time in the gay community as the "death-saturated culture."[4]

Today, the epidemiology of HIV disease remains the same as it has always been; in the United States, AIDS is still primarily an urban phenomenon. In medium-sized and smaller cities, the number of people infected and the number of deaths due to HIV is lower.[5] But seropositive individuals in smaller urban and rural areas and those who care for them and mourn their loss face an added burden. Medical knowledge and availability of services are more limited, while the prevalence of prejudice toward the disease may be greater. Many must cope with the disease and their grief in isolation.

In April 1996, as news of the promise of combination therapy was documented in the news media, the Names Project Foundation sponsored a display of the AIDS Memorial Quilt in Washington, D.C. The quilt completely covered the Washington mall, representing more than 70,000 individuals lost to HIV disease. For the first time, the president of the United States publicly viewed the quilt amidst an outpouring of sympathy from most sectors of the American public. By March of 1997, at the fourth conference on Human Retroviruses and Opportunistic Infections, there were optimistic reports on dramatic benefits from the use of triple-drug combinations, including protease inhibitors and other antiviral medications. The media was replete with stories of people with HIV who, once considered in the terminal phase of disease, had regained their strength and health.

Today, concerns about access to care, adherence to treatment regimens, and treatment failure temper earlier optimism. At the same time, there is a rise of new infections and a trend among younger people to disregard AIDS prevention messages. The epidemic is far from over.

Learning from History: Is AIDS Bereavement Unique?

In what has been described as a "culture of mourning," people associated with those groups most affected by HIV disease routinely experience chronic loss. As of 1994, 60 percent of gay men were losing at least one person a year to AIDS, and one-third of these bereaved individuals described multiple loss of family, friends, and neighbors.[6] This presents individuals in groups hardest hit by the epidemic with a dilemma: on one hand, being active in these communities can provide individuals with support in facing the epidemic; on the other hand, such community integration increases the risk that the individual will experience multiple loss.

Despite new medical treatments that have prolonged the lives and decreased the number of deaths from HIV disease, deaths continue to occur. The epidemic of HIV-related grief has slowed but is far from over. Even with a 12 percent decline in HIV mortality in the United States in 1996, 22,000 Americans died of AIDS in the first six months of that year.[7]

The research literature supports the conclusion that people facing AIDS bereavement present both similarities and differences when compared to people facing other types of grief. For example, a

New York study conducted early in the epidemic found that people grieving both HIV-related losses and other types of losses experienced similar grief symptoms including numbness, denial, and preoccupation with the deceased.[8] A more recent study compared AIDS bereavement versus cancer bereavement within the first three months after a loss.[9] Specifically, mourners in these two groups were similar in terms of the intensity of grief, and the existence of traumatic stress, grief-related depression symptoms, and general psychiatric symptoms, including anxiety, depression, somatic symptoms, and social dysfunction. They differed in that AIDS mourners reported lower levels of social support in response to bereavement and a greater number of losses. They were more likely to hide the cause of death from others and reported more support from friends than from family. In addition, some AIDS-bereaved individuals reported increased levels of rejection from other people.

In contrast to most life-threatening diseases, HIV disease has had an impact on disproportionate numbers of young and middle-aged people. Such premature death may be expected to increase the risk of prolonged or pathological grief reactions in loved ones.[10] In addition, the stigma associated with AIDS, homosexuality, and substance abuse may prevent some people from seeking support from community resources. The likelihood of multiple and chronic losses due to the epidemic further increases the burden for people with the disease and those who care for and mourn them. Finally, given that these losses exist within the context of an epidemic, a sizable group of caregivers and mourners are HIV-infected and struggle to cope with their own health concerns at the same time as they minister to others. Thus, the history of HIV is a history of loss, of deferred mourning and resolution of grief, and of balancing self-care and care for others – factors all surfacing in the context of stigma and, for many, isolation.

The Cultural Context of Mourning

AIDS mourners come from all walks of life and backgrounds. An understanding of cultural differences, and differences of class, gender, and sexual orientation is crucial to the development of competent approaches that are requisite for all counseling responses to bereavement. Given the level of HIV-related stigma – particularly as it focuses on traditionally stigmatized groups – an appreciation of culture beyond stereotypes is especially important.

Mindy Thompson Fullilove writes, "Stereotypes replace an understanding of the individual with imaginary characteristics of the group to which the individual belongs. Stereotypes concretize images of groups, preventing exploration of a complex reality. Stereotypes applied to individuals in therapy effectively block exploration of the self."[11] Fullilove also warns against simplistic approaches to cultural sensitivity that provide "factoid" snapshots of complex cultural phenomena. Such brief descriptions fail to embody the diversity within a culture and thus cannot be applied to individuals. In Fullilove's words, "Cultures are created and sustained by the interaction of groups in a particular place at a particular time. The beliefs of the group may govern the actions of the individual, but they cannot be assumed to define the individual."[11]

In exploring cultural differences among mourners, clinicians need to ask clients for clarification rather than to make assumptions. In general, counselors must ascertain how clients' specific concerns relate to their larger cultural belief system and reflect cultural norms. In helping AIDS mourners, clinicians need to inquire about clients' personal and culturally based beliefs about AIDS, death, and mourning, and identify the culturally based institutions and strategies clients use to cope with these issues.

The Cultural Construction of Death and Mourning

To comprehend cultural differences related to death and mourning, it is important to keep in mind the distinction between mourning and grief. Grief is an individual's underlying emotional response to loss, while mourning denotes actions and expressions of grief, which often reflect the customs of a person's culture. Further, it is useful to understand both the prevailing beliefs and customs within a culture and to appreciate the individual variance within that culture.

In her description of death in American culture, Kathy Charmatz emphasizes the prevailing Protestant ethic in the United States, starting from a focus on individual achievement, self-sufficiency, privatism, and hard work.[12] She states that there is a tendency to view death as a problem, which suggests that there are solutions to it. These solutions are typically of a technical nature, whether they require medical or psychotherapeutic responses. Further, given the tendency toward the smaller nuclear families, mourners have fewer people to turn to in times of loss.

Anthropologists Peter Metcalf and Richard Huntington have studied mourning rituals in a variety of cultures. In their book, *Celebrations of Death,* they explain that to understand mourning cross culturally, "We can assume neither the universality of particular modes of feeling nor that similar signs of emotion correspond to the same underlying sentiments in different cultures."[13] The emotional response to death is typically consistent with a culture's construction of what comes after death. While throughout the world, death is generally a time for the expression of strong emotional response – such as crying and breast-beating – for some cultures burials are joyful occasions requiring dancing and flirting. For example, in Java, mortality does not seem to hold any great terror, and the Javanese discuss death with little show of anxiety. In part, this calm is due to a pervasive fatalism about dying. It is all in the hands of God. Death is seen as a good state, empty of desire and striving. Youngsters who openly express sorrow are taught to regain composure.[13]

Similarly, according to Metcalf and Huntington, mourning practices cannot be explained simply as an outgrowth of an individual's psychological need to work through grief, release aggression, break ties with the deceased, or complete any other putative universal psychic process. They propose that, "Whatever mental adjustments the individual needs to make in the face of death, he or she must accomplish as best they can through or around such rituals as society provides. No doubt, the rites frequently aid adjustment. But we have no reason to believe that they do not obstruct it with equal frequency."[13]

Given the breadth of the HIV epidemic, it is no surprise that the responses to HIV-related deaths are varied, both in this country and abroad. Nonetheless the similarities among grieving individuals from different cultures are also striking. In a fascinating discussion of AIDS bereavement in Uganda, Janet Seeley and Ellen Kajura report: "The fact that there is no cure for AIDS has unwittingly programmed the minds of people to become uncommonly tolerant of death. Even the most robust and promising of young Africans may accept as inevitable that their deaths are imminent."[14] While this fatalist attitude toward death is consistent with a traditional view in that culture of predestination and a strong belief in survival after death, Seeley and Kajura observe that mourning practices have shifted since the AIDS epidemic. Traditionally, Ugandans observed a lengthy period of mourning: two to six months for a chief and a month for an ordinary male household head. Today, however, the amount of time spent mourning has decreased considerably, largely because the great number of deaths place extra burdens on the ability to financially support one's family. At the same time, Seeley and Kajura found that villagers were still concerned about fulfilling customary mourning obligations to the dead person. They also described intense grief among many survivors, who spoke of their loneliness and the sadness they felt for relatives who died young and "were not able to see any reward for their hard work."

Common to the AIDS experience worldwide, Seeley and Kajura found that economic, social, and political factors impinge upon the way people react to HIV infection and death. For example, stigma leads many Ugandans to try to disassociate themselves from the disease when a family member or neighbor has died. The cause of death is rarely acknowledged during funerals, and sometimes people even disown their kin after the death and refuse any show of condolence. This ethnographic example clearly suggests the complexity of the effects of AIDS on mourning within a cultural context. Specifically, it demonstrates the interplay between mourning customs and the responses of individuals to the deaths within the AIDS epidemic.

AIDS Bereavement Institutions and Customs

Many of the early institutions associated with HIV disease centered within the gay and lesbian community and focused primarily on the needs of that community. As the epidemic spread into other groups, some of these early institutions broadened their scope to include others. At the same time, new institutions were spawned either with broader focus or specifically addressing the needs of other communities. However, not all communities with high HIV-related prevalence have been eager to address the issue.

In a review of HIV care in African American communities, Larry Gant suggests that many African Americans have been reluctant to use HIV services and to openly confront the issue of AIDS within their community.[15] He states that, "African Americans have had mixed results in their use of HIV-specific support structures without the loss of personal or cultural integrity." He suggests that compared to gay white men, African Americans seek informal, nonprofessional, noncredentialed, nonbureaucratic helpers for problems of low to moderate severity, and seek professional support only when problems escalate to a critical stage, for example, in the context of a nervous breakdown or extreme physical illness.

Another reason Gant cites for the reluctance of many nongay individuals to use HIV services is the fear of further stigmatization. For example, African Americans, recent immigrants, and substance users, already marginalized by society, may be hesitant to participate in an HIV-identified program for fear that they may be further identified as an outsider or may be wrongly identified as homosexual. On a more positive note, many nongay people confronting losses due to AIDS may choose pre-existing resources within their communities – such as family or church – to cope with the burdens of AIDS and its losses.

The reliance of many gay men on community-based HIV-oriented institutions, rather than on family and religious institutions, may represent a cultural phenomenon more specific to that community alone. This phenomenon may be most pronounced in larger urban areas that serve as migration centers for gay men and lesbians fleeing the prejudice of their home towns. Many gay men in mourning are separated from family and from childhood religious communities. Michael Shernoff, coining the term "gay widower" to describe gay men who have survived the death of a partner, noted the lack of a literature depicting the experience of these men. In a collection of essays by gay men describing their experiences of coping with the death of a partner, Shernoff says, "When a gay man's partner dies, his trauma is often exacerbated by the lack of mainstream culture's recognition of his relationship, his loss, and being a widower."[16,17]

To combat this sense of isolation and devaluation, gay men and lesbians have created various activities to memorialize HIV-related deaths, reflecting cultural attitudes within that community and including ritual or ceremony to provide structure for their grief. Through traditional and personalized rituals or ceremonies, mourners seek to combat the sense of helplessness that often accompanies grief and to find a legitimate form to express strong grief-related emotions. Community ceremonies, for example, candlelight marches, "celebrations of life," and memorial services, invite participants to surrender their individuality and become immersed in a cause larger than themselves, thus decreasing alienation. Often these newer forms of mourning rituals combine political, spiritual, and personal symbols with humor. While these ceremonies may or may not include the families of origin of the deceased, a common theme is the reaffirmation of the legitimacy of being gay.

Finding Personal Meaning in AIDS Mourning

On reflecting upon the death of a loved one, each mourner must ask, "What specific meaning does this death have for me?" For some, the meaning is obvious, immediate, and concrete. The loss, especially of a life partner or a spouse, raises immediate questions such as, "How will I handle aspects of our shared life that had been handled by my partner?" As a person moves from caregiver to mourner, life reverts in some ways back to pre-caretaking days, yet this is a lonely return reflective of a loss. This shift not only concerns tasks, but also identity: "Who am I now that I am alone?" While the challenges of these practical questions are great and play a large role in determining whether a person will adapt adequately to the loss, more abstract questions may also affect the emotional well-being of the mourner. Questions such as "Why did this happen?" and "What does this loss say about the meaning of life?" may cause some mourners even more stress than specific life problems.

Loss and World View

The search for meaning in bereavement does not begin at the time of death. Each mourner comes to bereavement with previously held beliefs and values, and these may undergo change throughout the course of the loved one's illness. To a large extent, the way a person understands the loss is affected by the nature of the specific relationship mourned, the view held by the mourner regarding relationships in general, and broader beliefs about the nature of the world. AIDS mourners may assign idiosyncratic meanings to the illness and how it is transmitted, sometimes resulting in negative evaluations that get projected on people most likely to contract the disease.

According to Camille Wortman and her colleagues, one group of mourners at risk for bereavement distress are those for whom the loss cannot be incorporated into their philosophical perspective of the world.[18] For these individuals, the loss shatters their world view, that is, the interwoven system of beliefs, assumptions, and expectations that provide a sense of coherence and meaning. Wortman found her subjects varied in terms of their view of the world as: predictable and orderly versus random, safe versus dangerous, benevolent versus malevolent, controllable versus uncontrollable, fair versus unfair, and trustworthy versus untrustworthy. She also found that people may be fatalistic, seeing all things as part of a larger plan; they may believe that people get what they earn or deserve, either on this earth or in the afterlife; or they may view the world as a random universe or a "jungle" where things happen without purpose.

When confronted by a loss inconsistent with their world views, some mourners may adopt a new world view that facilitates subsequent coping efforts. Others, however, may live permanently with unresolved conflict, typically leading them to "give up on the world" and hold back from future relationships. Those individuals, who initially viewed the world as controllable, predictable, and safe, may be particularly vulnerable to uncontrollable life events such as a death of a spouse. Thus, unlike some bereavement researchers who found negative bereavement consequences to be due primarily to unsatisfying and ambivalent relationships, Wortman identified another group at risk: those with the highest self-esteem, the highest feelings of mastery, the greatest intellectual resources, and the most financial resources. In line with her hypothesis of "shattered meaning," it makes sense that the most emotionally stable individuals and those with the best relationships have the most to lose and may be at higher risk for complicated grieving.

Existential psychotherapist Irvin Yalom writes that, "Human beings seem to require meaning. To live without meaning, values, or ideals seems to provoke considerable distress."[19] He refers to Victor Frankl's observations that in the German concentration camps, the individual with no sense of meaning was unlikely to survive. Yalom divides the search for meaning into two interrelated questions: "What is the meaning of life?" and, "What is the meaning of my life?" He proposes that the former is an inquiry into cosmic meaning, a question of whether life fits into some overall coherent pattern. The latter is focused on secular meaning, a question of whether life has some purpose or function to be fulfilled, some overriding goal or goals to which a person can apply him or herself.[19]

Cosmic Meaning

Mourners throughout time and around the world have turned to religion to find meaning and comfort after the loss of a loved one.

According to Yalom, "Within the Western world, the Judeo-Christian religious tradition has offered a comprehensive meaning-schema based upon the principle that the world and human life are part of a divinely ordained plan."[19] More recently, in some parts of the world, newer forms of religious thought and practices – referred to as "New Age" or simply as "spirituality" – have become popular. These philosophical and religious paths tend to be more individualized and combine aspects of both Western and Eastern points of view.

In her doctoral dissertation, Claire Costello – using data collected by Susan Nolen-Hoeksema and her colleagues at Stanford – studied the role of religion and philosophical beliefs in coping with an HIV-related death.[20] Her study group consisted of 95 AIDS mourners – gay male friends and partners and nongay family members. She found that a stable and consistent match between a person's religious, spiritual, or philosophical beliefs and behaviors created a stress buffer in AIDS bereavement. That is, it appears that the most important factor determining how a person copes with an AIDS death is not whether a person considers him or herself religious, spiritual, or agnostic, but whether his or her philosophy and actions are consistent.

Several findings led Costello to the conclusion that consistency of philosophy and action is the necessary ingredient for reducing stress in bereavement. First, "agnostic" subjects did as well with AIDS bereavement as "religious" subjects. Second, subjects who identified themselves as "religious" or "spiritual" and who frequently participated in religious or spiritual activities coped better than those who did not. Specifically, those individuals who not only had religious or spiritual beliefs but also practiced those beliefs through prayer or meditation fared better than those who claimed a religious affiliation but did not actively participate in their faith. Third, in an almost humorous outcome: the group of AIDS mourners in her study who were most depressed and coped least effectively was "agnostics who prayed."

Interestingly, in Costello's sample – contrary to expectation – gay subjects were as likely to consider themselves as "religious" as nongay subjects and were more likely to consider themselves "religious" than "spiritual." Another unexpected finding was that gay partners and friends, more often than family members, were able to use the support of churches to help them with their HIV-related bereavement. This may speak to the hesitancy on the part of some nongay individuals to be open about the AIDS-related nature of their loss in traditional religious venues.

Costello also found that those respondents who reported a sense of personal growth from their bereavement experience were less likely to suffer destructive rumination. She reported typical statements of personal meaning from these respondents. One person told the interviewer, "I discovered why I was put on this earth, I take care of people." Another said, "I've learned – [am] beginning to learn – more about myself. I'm proud of myself for handling things the way I did." A third said, "It's made me more conscious every day, of everything, oh that flowers are beautiful . . . ." Costello findings are clearly consistent with Wortman's notion that religious and philosophical beliefs can protect a bereaved person from distress by helping him or her incorporate loss into a world view.[18]

There are obvious limitations to empirical studies of phenomena as complex and subtle as religious beliefs and actions. Even so, an important message does seem to come through in Costello's work: finding religious or philosophical meaning in the death of a loved one can assist the bereavement process. The following statement by the gay widower Townsand Price-Spratlen demonstrates how mourning the loss of his former lover helped him find spiritual meaning in his life.

> *Tony's passing has transformed my life by changing my view of, and relationship toward, expressions of faith and other spiritual celebrations. His passing teaches me that it is possible to live joyously, healthfully, and lovingly, and any laughter shared is not disrespecting memories tinged with sadness.*[21]

Secular Meaning

Secular humans face the task of finding some direction to life without an external beacon.[19] Fortunately for those who are not religiously inclined, according to Costello's findings, having a consistent secular philosophy appears to be as beneficial as having a religious one in combating the stress of mourning. Most existential philosophy asserts – as did Camus and Sartre – that human beings must invent their own meaning, rather than discover God's or nature's meaning, and then commit fully to fulfilling that meaning.[19]

Irvin Yalom outlines six secular activities that provide human beings with a sense of purpose in their lives. These activities are also frequently seen among HIV mourners. The first two activities – altruism and dedicating oneself to a cause – are hallmarks of HIV activism. A remarkable legacy of community organizations exists as a result of the hard work of those who care about combating the AIDS epidemic. The third – finding a creative outlet – has been demonstrated throughout the epidemic. Whether manifested as a quilt panel, a comedy act, or a scientific discovery, HIV has spawned an immense number of creative projects.

Yalom's fourth secular activity is to find a hedonistic solution: "The purpose of life is simply to live fully, to retain one's sense of astonishment at the miracle of life, to plunge oneself into the natural rhythm of life, to search for pleasure in the deepest possible sense." The hedonist takes a page from the human potential movement of the 1970s and works to live in the present or as the mantra of that time would have it, "Be here now." A more uproarious variation on this theme is the *Auntie Mame* posture seen among some vivacious drag performers who continually exhort us to "Live, live, live!"

Yalom's last two activities – self-actualization and self-transcendence – are closest to secular "religions" and embody a humanistic view. As articulated by Abraham Maslow, self-actualization holds that a person has within him or herself a proclivity toward growth, a unity of personality, and an inherent blueprint consisting of a unique set of characteristics and a drive to express them. The highest urges of an individual, once his or her more basic needs are met, are for knowledge, insight, and wisdom. Furthermore, those actualized individuals have an aesthetic need for symmetry, congruence, integration, beauty, meditation, creativity, and harmony. Every person lives to fulfill his or her potential.

Where self-actualization and hedonism are concerned with the self, self-transcendence reflects some basic craving to go beyond one's self-interest and to strive toward something or someone outside or "above" oneself.[19] For some moral philosophers the notion of self-actualization is disturbing in its self-focus. For example, Victor Frankl believed that excessive concern with self-expression and self-actualization thwarts the search for genuine meaning. He said the inability to focus on the needs of others blocks an individual's desire for intimacy. While receding from others may become attractive during mourning and may even be beneficial for a period, it must be reconsidered over time.[19]

A developmental psychology perspective adds to this discussion of self-actualization and self-transcendence. According to Erik Erikson, there is a gradual evolution of meanings throughout a person's life cycle.[19] In adolescence and early and middle adulthood, people place primary concern on themselves as they struggle to establish stable identities, to develop intimate relationships, and to achieve a sense of mastery in their professional endeavors. Unless they fail to negotiate an earlier developmental task, people in their forties and fifties pass into a stage where they find meaning in self-transcendent ventures. Erikson called this stage "generativity," with its goal being establishing and guiding the next generation; and generativity may take the form of specific concern for one's progeny or more broadly for the care of the species.

Christopher Mead, an American Jungian analyst living in the Netherlands, points out that HIV disease interferes with the normal psychological development of seropositive people and those who care for them, most of whom are between 20 years old and 39 years old.[22] According to Mead, HIV disease requires these young people to take on the developmental tasks of old age at a time when they often lack the experience to cope with these issues. The psyche unprepared for this responsibility is placed in crisis. Crisis brings with it the possibility of both psychological growth and destruction. If individuals in this situation do not develop conscious or unconscious solutions to these challenges, they face the danger of developing psychological problems such as the re-emergence of old conflicts regarding sexual orientation. On the other hand, those with the requisite psychological resources may find wisdom far beyond their years.

True Story Two: A Family Finds Meaning within Its Grief

Below is the second true story in this monograph. It illustrates a family's personal growth through its search for meaning through creativity, community involvement, and remembrance.

This is my story about our family's experience before and after the death of our son Vincent Joseph Sansevero, III. Vinny died May 5, 1995, at the very young age of 34. He faced his failing health with admirable acceptance and bravery; I never accepted that he was dying – not even on the way to the hospital in the ambulance. As I look back, I understand that in many ways, Vinny was trying to prepare me for his death. We all felt his suffering, and he knew his family would have gone to the end of the earth for him. The determination and strength that became so much part of his life as he faced eternity was inspirationally powerful.

Our family watched Vinny live with AIDS as everything was taken away from him – his health, his achievements, his life. We watched him quickly turn from perfect health to a sick, frail, suffering young man. Although we will never recover from his loss, making his panel for the AIDS Memorial Quilt helped me to tell his story and become an advocate for AIDS education.

I worked on Vinny's panel with family and friends for one year. It stayed on our dining room table the entire time it was being created. It was hard for me to give it up. A dear friend told me that it had to leave the house so that many people would learn about Vinny's life. The panel left Connecticut to be incorporated into the Quilt in May of '96. That October the entire family went to Washington, D.C. to view the Quilt in its entirety, in the presence of thousands of people displaying heartfelt empathy with tears and silence; it was a remarkable experience that brought all of us closer.

When the Quilt was displayed in Connecticut last year, I gave a ten-minute presentation at each of four high schools. I feel that I am keeping Vinny's memory alive by telling his story as well as bringing the realities of AIDS to young people. The following are some thoughts from Vinny's sister Christine: "I am filled with sorrow and tears over the loss of someone so close to my heart, my older brother. I do not know why this had to happen to him . . . and to us. He achieved so much in such a short period of time and certainly had much left to do. I think of Vinny every day and miss him terribly. As a family we talk about him all the time with laughter and tears. This is part of our responsibility. Vinny will not be forgotten and will continue to make a difference in the world through us. The pain of his absence will never subside, but neither will the memory of his hopes, dreams, and love.[23]

The Psychology of Grief

Over the years, psychological theory and observations pertaining to the nature of grief have been grounded in clinical experience, empirical findings with clinical and nonclinical populations, and naturalistic observations. Underlying each attempt to understand the nature of grief is an explicit or implicit psychological theory. Broadly speaking, two theoretical orientations have been most widely applied to the study of bereavement: psychodynamic and cognitive.

Psychodynamic theories have generally attempted to understand the underlying conscious and unconscious processes that mediate the grief process. Cognitive-behavioral theories have been more concerned with factors related to stress and coping that affect bereavement distress. This monograph attempts to synthesize these two approaches into a comprehensive clinical model. Psychodynamic observations – derived largely from the work of John Bowlby, J. William Worden, and Mardi Horowitz – underlie the following discussion of the course of grief; cognitively based research informs the analysis of risk factors for bereavement distress.

The origins of the psychological study of bereavement are usually traced to Freud's observations on mourning and melancholia. While the terms mourning and melancholia are used differently today, Freud's description of what we now term grief – the emotional response to loss – and its differentiation from depression remain relevant to modern psychological views of bereavement. According to Freud:

> *Mourning [grief] is the profoundly painful dejection, cessation of interest in the outside world, loss of the capacity to love, inhibition of all activity. . . . It is really only because we know so well how to explain it that this attitude does not seem to us pathological. Melancholia, on the other hand, shares the above features but also includes a lowering of self-regarding feelings to a degree that finds utterance in self-reproaches and self-revilings, and culminates in a delusional expectation of punishment.*[24]

In comforting those suffering grief, we often say that "Time heals all wounds," or that "Mourning cannot be rushed." But how long is it normal to grieve? There is little agreement among experts regarding the normal length of grief, yet grief symptoms do tend to diminish over time. Some studies that have followed the bereaved longitudinally have found that many people are still actively grieving after thirteen months.[25] Even ten years after the loss, researchers have observed in bereaved people, who were otherwise functioning well, milder grief symptoms such as often thinking, dreaming, or missing a loved one and responding to reminders of him or her by crying or experiencing distress.[26] Similarly, research on AIDS bereavement has found that although for most people symptoms of grief and depression significantly diminish over time, a subgroup of AIDS mourners continue to suffer severely even a year-and-a-half after the death of a loved one.[27,28]

Given that time alone is not an adequate indicator of grief resolution, are there other ways of determining whether mourning is going well or not? Several psychodynamically oriented authors have described grief as a process that can be understood in terms of phases or tasks. While these models are helpful in educating mourners as to what to expect during the process of grief and in identifying those mourners who are somehow blocked in resolving their grief, several cautions apply to these findings. First, Stephen Shuchter and Sidney Zisook admonish that, "Grief is not a linear process with concrete boundaries, but rather a composite of overlapping, fluid phases that vary from person to person."[29] Second, Camille Wortman's research indicates that a sizable minority of mourners is able to manage the course of grief with little or no bereavement distress.[18]

John Bowlby: Four Phases of Grief

In the 1960s, John Bowlby published his monumental three-volume collection entitled *Attachment, Separation, and Loss*.[30] By studying the reactions of both young children and primates separated from their mother figure, Bowlby developed a comprehensive theory of the process of attachment formation and the psychological reaction to separation and loss. His theory added to prevailing psychoanalytic observations of grief, observations drawn from ethology (the study of behavior patterns in animals), control theory, cognitive psychology, and cybernetics.

Bowlby suggests that over the course of weeks and months, bereaved individuals typically move through a succession of four phases. These phases overlap and individuals may oscillate back and forth between any two. The four phases are: shock and numbing; yearning and searching; disorganization and despair; and greater or lesser degrees of reorganization.[30] Bowlby believes that *complicated grief*, a concept that is crucial to clinical practice, is best understood as an exaggeration or distortion of the normal process of grieving. Consistent with this definition, this monograph defines *uncomplicat-*

ed grief as the adequate management of the grief process in which the mourner successfully moves through the phases and tasks of mourning consistent with his or her own values and cultural norms.

Phase of Shock and Numbing

According to Bowlby, the initial reaction to the death of a loved one is shock. Given that most AIDS deaths come after an extended period of severe physical decline, they are frequently expected. Even so, most AIDS mourners experience some form of early emotional withdrawal, a mixture of relief and loss, and sometimes, surprise. Among primary caregivers, the initial period of shock and numbing is typically exacerbated by sheer exhaustion from the overwhelming demands of caring for a terminally ill person. This is especially true for those caregivers who have received limited emotional or practical support from others. For a time shortly after the death, some mourners may carry on their activities as if nothing has happened. This approach typically falls away and grief-related anxiety and anger find their way to the surface.

Phase of Yearning and Searching

Once the bereaved registers the reality of the loss, often a period of intense pining begins. During this time, the mourner may experience a great restlessness, insomnia, and preoccupation with thoughts of the lost loved one. Some mourners have the sense of actual presence, a marked tendency to interpret sounds as indicating that the lost person is returning. It is not uncommon to have vivid dreams of the lost loved one still alive and well, accompanied by corresponding desolation upon waking.

Another common element in the second phase of mourning is anger. Similar to the children described by Bowlby who were separated from their mothers, adult mourners exhibit *protest* behaviors and efforts to recover the lost love. Anger is aroused both by those held responsible for the loss and by the frustrations of the fruitless search. In mourning that runs a healthy course, the urge to search and recover, often intense in the early weeks and months, tends to diminish gradually over time. As anger and anxiety related to both conscious or unconscious efforts to reunite dissipates, sadness and sorrow appear. Bowlby maintains that many of the features characteristic of complicated grief result from the active persistence of the urge to recover the lost loved one, an urge that tends to be expressed in a variety of disguised and distorted ways.

Phase of Disorganization and Despair and Phase of Reorganization

According to Bowlby, for mourning to have a favorable outcome, it appears to be necessary for a bereaved person to endure intense pining, more or less conscious searching, seemingly endless examination of how and why the loss occurred, and anger at anyone who might have been responsible – not sparing even the dead person. Once a mourner can accept the despair that none of these activities will bring back the lost love, he or she can gradually accept that the loss is permanent and that life must take new shape.

At this point many emotional and behavioral routines must be modified. Slowly, the old well-rehearsed patterns of daily living begin to change and the phase of reorganization begins. A great deal of vacillation occurs between disorganization and reorganization. Some aspects of life may be more easily altered: a person can find new people with whom to eat meals, and tasks around the house – formally allocated to the deceased – can be accomplished in other ways. Other aspects may take longer, with failed attempts along the way. This is especially true in terms of personal communication and affection, the more intimate aspects of life. Some mourners attempt to "replace" loved ones soon after the loss. While this occasionally works, most find that fleeing into a new relationships results in disappointment.

The timing of this phase of grief is largely dictated by personal values and cultural norms. Our culture expects grieving individuals to return to work within a week or two. Many gay men, whose relationships are not acknowledged at work, may be required to return even sooner. Even humane employers who may not expect mourners to be immediately at "full speed" assume that in a fairly short amount of time these employees will be able to perform up to expectations. Returning to dating or resuming intimate relationships is not so clearly defined in modern urban secular living. Long gone are ritualized periods of mourning. Such cultural guidance is especially lacking in the gay community, where norms for relationships are even less well-articulated than in American culture as a whole.

J. William Worden: the Four Tasks of Mourning

J. William Worden published his influential book *Grief Counseling and Grief Therapy* in 1982. Based largely on Bowlby's work on attachment and on empirical studies of spousal bereavement, Worden proposes four tasks of mourning that he suggests must be accomplished before mourning is complete.[31] Worden's concept of the tasks of mourning emphasizes intentional actions on the part of the mourner to complete the process rather than a resolution of grief occurring naturally over time. Worden's tasks are:

- To accept the reality of the loss;
- To experience the pain of grief;
- To adjust to an environment in which the deceased is missing;
- To withdraw emotional energy and reinvest it in another relationship.

A drawback to Worden's model is that it is based on his work with bereaved spouses. In particular, the fourth task – withdrawal of emotional energy and reinvesting in another relationship – is not appropriate for all mourners, for example, family members. To accommodate the challenge of mourning the irreplaceable loss of a child or a parent, the fourth task might be better conceptualized as "beginning or returning to avenues for personal growth and expression." This is nicely illustrated in the story of the Sansevero family, presented earlier in this chapter, who mourn the loss of their son and brother, Vinny.

On the other hand, the notion of tasks of grief has an advantage over the idea of phases, because tasks offer active guidance toward behavioral change. Having a positive focus and direction for managing grief can be enormously comforting to mourners. For this reason, explaining Worden's tasks of grief is often helpful in bereavement education for individual clients or within bereavement education group formats.

Mardi Horowitz: Psychological Mediation of Grief

Mardi Horowitz is another psychodynamically oriented bereavement researcher who proposes a phase model of grief. While Bowlby's understanding of how we adapt to loss is based on attachment theory, Horowitz's view of bereavement is grounded primarily in theories of stress and trauma. According to his model, in the aftermath of any stressful life event, certain processes must occur to facilitate assimilation, accommodation, and healthy resumption of living.[32] An individual's complex psychological reaction to loss incorporates elements of both the stressful event and the individual's pre-existing personality, including both conscious and unconscious mechanisms.

Like Bowlby, Horowitz integrates aspects of both psychodynamic and cognitive psychology into his model. Horowitz suggests that in order to cope adequately with an extreme stressor, an individual must resolve the personal meaning of the traumatic event. In order to return to pretraumatic levels of functioning, this resolution must include coming to terms with the implications it has for one's interpersonal relationships, one's self-image, and one's behavior. People tend to have characteristic ways of reacting to stress, for example, some respond with turbulent emotions while others stifle their feelings.

Drawing from the cognitive psychology principles of Jean Piaget, Horowitz uses the construct of *person schemata* to describe how people view themselves and others and how this view guides the collection and storage of information and directs their actions. For example in bereavement, when individuals experience a death of a loved one, they are forced to modify their schemata, to revise their core models of themselves, their role relationships, and their future plans. Upon hearing of the death of her husband, a woman must somehow change her view of herself and incorporate this information. Does she see herself once again as a "single person" or does she view herself as a "widow"? What are the implications of these changes? This rearrangement of person schemata takes time, and according to Horowitz, some of the disorientation seen in mourning is related to this reorganization process.

An important aspect of Horowitz's work, which is drawn from his psychoanalytic background, is his description of conscious and unconscious mechanisms to modulate impulses, ideas, and feelings. Perhaps Horowitz's greatest contribution to bereavement theory lies in his observations and explanations of a typical pattern for mourners: that is the vacillation between times of cognitive and emotional intrusion and times of psychological suppression of these disturbing thoughts and emotions. The extent to which a person allows thoughts, memories, or emotions to emerge into consciousness depends on the nature and effectiveness of internal control mechanisms. In healthy responses to bereavement, the mourner is able more or less to accommodate both states of emotional arousal and emotional withdrawal, until grief is "worked through." (Some writers use the metaphor of grief metabolism to describe this process.) In grief that has gone awry, the modulation of these states is faulty, characterized by either emotional overwhelm or extreme avoidance, sometimes referred to as psychic numbing.

Horowitz incorporated the concept of the psychological mediation of grief in his five-phase model, which includes: outcry, denial, intrusions, working-through, and completion. This model helps clinicians understand the underlying mechanisms of grief, and better differentiate normal grief from its complications.

Susan Folkman: Coping with the Stress of Grief

Whereas psychodynamic models of bereavement emphasize an underlying grief process expressed as stages or phases, cognitive models focus on mourner burden and the cognitive and behavioral skills needed to cope with these burdens. Susan Folkman and her colleagues at the Center for AIDS Prevention Studies at the University of California San Francisco have applied cognitive psychology theories of stress and coping to the understanding of both general and HIV-related bereavement. Folkman's framework views the loss of a loved one as a stressful event, that is, "one that involves a relationship between the individual and the environment that is appraised by the individual as personally meaningful and as taxing to personal resources."[27] In this view, loss causes stress when an individual perceives that the demands placed upon him or her by the loss, outweigh the resources that he or she has to cope with the situation.[27,33]

A key concept in stress and coping theory is *appraisal.* Appraisal refers to the cognitive evaluative process that imbues a situation or event with meaning regarding an individual's well-being.[34] Appraisal can be separated into those perceptions that are concerned with the recognition that an individual is in jeopardy (appraisal of what is at stake) and those that are concerned primarily with the evaluation of the availability of resources for managing potential or actual harm. An individual may appraise an event as irrelevant, a threat, or an indication that some harm or loss has already occurred. On the other hand, individuals may find an event or situation to be a challenge, suggesting that the individual perceives a level of danger, but estimates that he or she has the where-with-all to cope with the danger. In order to cope effectively with a stressful situation, people must accurately appraise the nature and extent of the threat and, likewise, the resources available to them.

The second core concept in Folkman's model is *coping*. Coping is a process by which the individual changes cognitive or behavioral responses to manage the specific demands that are appraised as stressful. Coping has two major functions: to manage or change the problem that is causing the distress (problem-focused coping) and to regulate emotional responses to the problem (emotion-focused coping).[35] For example, the stress caused by financial concerns is best handled by taking constructive action to reduce spending, while the stress caused by waiting for test results requires managing the emotional reactions to an event outside one's control. Effective coping requires that the individual accurately appraise a stressful situation to determine which form of coping is appropriate and then competently apply the requisite forms of coping. Of course, many stresses encountered in real life require both problem-solving and emotion-focused coping strategies.[34]

Using the cognitive theory of stress and coping, Folkman and her colleagues developed the UCSF Coping Project, a large longitudinal investigation of HIV caregiving and bereavement. They described the stress of HIV caregiving as follows: "Providing care to a partner with advanced HIV disease constitutes a chronically stressful condition that is punctuated by specific stressful events related to the day-to-day demands of caregiving and approaching bereavement."[24]

In their study, the researchers collected data between 1990 and 1994 from 314 gay men, 253 caregiving partners of men with HIV disease, and 61 HIV-positive men in primary relationships with healthy partners. The researchers defined a caregiver as a man who identified as gay and was in a committed relationship with a partner who needed assistance with at least two instrumental tasks of daily living. As a premise of their study, the researchers hypothesized that the psychological well-being of individuals who serve as caregivers and then suffer the loss of their partners depended on the following appraisal and coping skills:

- The activation of personally meaningful beliefs and goals;
- The revision of untenable beliefs and goals, and the construction of concrete plans for the future;
- The experience of positive emotions and successful goal out-

comes in the recounting of past events associated with caregiving and the partner.

Discussion of this important large-scale study has been published in several articles and has included an analysis of the specific predictors of negative bereavement outcomes and strategies for enhancing coping among AIDS mourners.[27,35] Predictors of bereavement distress fall into roughly two categories: bereavement burdens (stressors faced by mourners) and coping skills to manage these burdens. Thus, to predict whether a mourner will develop negative bereavement outcomes, such as clinical depression, one must understand both the amount of burdens he or she faces above and beyond the death, as well as his or her level of skill in managing stress. The UCSF Coping Project has developed and evaluated specific strategies to reduce bereavement burden and increase coping skills. These interventions will be discussed further in Chapter Three.

Conclusion: Toward an Integrated Model of AIDS Bereavement

This chapter has cataloged the fundamental factors that influence AIDS bereavement. It has outlined the relationship between bereavement and the history of the epidemic, identifying the historical forces of stigma and isolation, and it has highlighted the sheer numbers of deaths that have accumulated over time. It has defined the role of culture and custom in determining individual responses to death, mourning, and bereavement, suggesting that cultural conceptions of death and mourning are varied, that these conceptions have a significant effect on the response to loss, and that while culture is part of the larger societal context, a provider's unchecked assumptions about culture and custom can sabotage effective counseling.

The second half of this chapter has identified the philosophical and psychological phenomena that operate on a more individual level as clients strive to find meaning and cope with loss. The philosophical aspect relates primarily to the ways in which a person comprehends secular or spiritual meaning in life, death, and grief. The psychological aspect relates to the ways in which a person proceeds through the grieving process, resolving grief, and coping or failing to cope with loss.

These four areas of influence combine to inform the Integrative

Model of AIDS Bereavement proposed in the next two chapters of this monograph. The model encourages clinicians to take a cross-cultural, multidisciplinary approach to working with AIDS mourners. It provides structures for clinicians to assist clients to understand their grief and to find meaning in their experience. It incorporates aspects of both the cognitive and psychodynamic views of bereavement to enhance accurate assessment of bereavement distress by establishing criteria to discern normal from complicated grief. Further, based on a review of the stress and coping literature, the model compiles a list of risk factors for AIDS bereavement distress. In this way, the model assists clinicians in selecting interventions that best address the specific needs of AIDS mourners in managing their grief and resolving specific grief-related problems.

2

Clinical Assessment of AIDS Bereavement Distress

A central tenet of the Integrative Model of AIDS Bereavement is that bereavement distress is not a single entity. Therefore, effective treatment requires precise assessment in order to define and address a mourner's particular concerns. This chapter describes the assessment process, reviewing the types and levels of bereavement distress and detailing the tools necessary to recognize these levels and their effects.

To apply the Integrative Model, the clinician first considers whether a client is currently experiencing uncomplicated grief or complicated grief with or without co-existing clinical disorders. Next, the clinician reviews bereavement risk factors to determine the likelihood of a mourner developing bereavement complications in the future or – in a case where complicated grief already exists – exacerbating current bereavement distress. Applying these considerations, the Integrative Model proposes four types and levels of AIDS bereavement distress:

- Uncomplicated Grief;
- Uncomplicated Grief with Risk Factors;
- Complicated Grief without Clinical Disorder;
- Complicated Grief with Clinical Disorder.

Understanding these levels and their defining criteria prepares clinicians to provide the types of interventions that will be most helpful to clients. As discussed in Chapter One, the term *complicated grief* indicates that the normal course of grief has gone awry. Complicated grief is distinguished from uncomplicated grief by a disruption in the course of grief as characterized by:

> An atypical intensity (overly numbed or overly intrusive) or duration (absent or chronic) of grief symptoms (shock, yearning, searching, disorganization, despair), which leads to an unacceptable duration of functional impairment in critical areas of work and relations.

The term *risk factors* refers to predictors that are associated with negative bereavement outcomes.[1] The identification of specific risk factors for AIDS bereavement distress both signals the need for bereavement interventions and directs the clinician toward the appropriate type and focus of intervention. Knowledge of risk factors can also assist a wide range of helping professionals – such as clergy, teachers, medical providers – identify AIDS mourners who might benefit from further evaluation by a knowledgeable mental health professional. Working in a proactive manner, alert helping professionals can educate clients to their risk factors and early warning signs of complicated grief, so that they can seek help before more severe problems develop. Assessment of AIDS bereavement – including complicated grief, risk factors, or associated clinical disorder – requires clinicians to undertake a thorough history, including a history of the bereaved relationship (as it was before, during, and after the death), a standard diagnostic review of signs and symptoms of clinical disorder, and a survey of the number and magnitude of AIDS bereavement risk factors.

Distinguishing Complicated and Uncomplicated Grief

The distinction between uncomplicated grief and complicated grief is based largely on the subjective experience of the mourner, requiring the input and self-evaluation of each mourner regarding his or her experience of the grieving process. As noted in Chapter One, broad individual and cultural differences exist regarding expectations about the intensity and duration of grief. Clinicians need to be prepared to help clients examine whether the level of grief they experience is consistent with their personal values and the values of their cultures.

If a client labels his or her grief as a problem – if for example, it is "too little" or "too much" – clinicians must ascertain for whom it is a problem. In some cases, families or employers may feel that the grief is going on too long, while a mourner is content to continue to experience it. On the other hand, well-meaning counselors – basing care on the outmoded assumption that intense grief is requisite – may mistakenly communicate that a person should feel and express more grief than is necessary for that individual.

Beyond the subjective evaluation of grief, assessment should be based on well-grounded bereavement theory and research. The systematic differentiation between complicated and uncomplicated grief has received a great deal of theoretical and empirical attention in the past twenty years. Even so, there is no universally accepted diagnostic schema currently in place. For example, there is no diagnostic category for complicated grief in the *Diagnostic and Statistical Manual of Mental Disorders.*[36] While a consensus appears to be emerging, a great deal of work needs to be done to unify research and theory into a single set of criteria. The following description of the distinction between complicated and uncomplicated grief is a synthesis of the literature and focuses on disruptions in the course of grief, the role of functional impairment in complicating grief, and symptoms of complicated grief.

Disruptions in the Course of Grief

John Bowlby discusses two variants of complicated grief that incorporate the issues of duration and intensity of grief: *absent grief* and *chronic grief*. For Bowlby, the lack of a grief reaction after a significant loss often indicates that the normal course of grief has been blocked.[30] It is important to remember, however, that research has consistently shown that about 20 percent of mourners do not exhibit intense symptoms of grief, and this has no apparent negative effect on their future adaptation.[18,27] In these cases, the absence of grief may indicate that an individual was well-prepared for the loss, as in response to the long-expected death of an aged and gravely ill parent, or that the actual level of attachment with the deceased was minimal.[37]

At other times, however, the absence of grief is an indication of an impeded mourning process, usually stemming from psychological defenses, conscious or unconscious, such as denial or repression. In Bowlby's words, it is, "A brief phase of numbing we now know to be very common following bereavement; but we do not expect it to last more than a few days or perhaps a week. When it lasts for longer there is reason for unease; for example, we have seen how delay of a few weeks or months may presage chronic mourning."[30]

In some cases, it may be difficult to discern whether the lack of strong grief following a loss is pathological or within normal range. To aid in this distinction, Bowlby observed that in blocked or absent grief there are often "tell-tale signs" that the bereaved person has, in fact, been affected and that his or her mental equilibrium is disturbed. Blocked or absent grief is often seen in individuals with a high need for self-control, and who scorn sentiment and pride themselves on carrying on as though nothing has happened. While to the casual observer, these mourners may appear to be coping well, on closer examination they appear tense and driven, sometimes experiencing physical symptoms such as headaches, palpitations, insomnia, and nightmares. Often, these mourners manifest breakthrough emotions such as rage or depression, even though they do not attribute these to loss. Other avoidance signs may appear, for example, evasion of consolation and certain topics. Some mourners compulsively work or take care of others.

Over time, many who have avoided mourning an important loss may express a generalized dissatisfaction with their lives. Bowlby noted that at some point over the course of mourning, many of these individuals develop some form of depression. He outlined several events that may precipitate depression in such cases: an anniversary of the death that has not been mourned; another loss; the birthday of a child reaching the same age as a loved one who has died; or the loss of someone who was the object of compulsive caregiving.

According to Bowlby, chronic grief involves the undesired persistence of grief reactions, including shock, yearning, searching, disorganization, and despair. In the most severe form of chronic mourning, painful memories and thoughts intrude into consciousness and interrupt occupational and social functioning. Although chronic grief often is unremitting, it is not unusual for chronic mourners to vacillate between periods of absent and acute grief.

For Bowlby, chronic mourning is defined not only by the duration of grief, but also by subtle differences in the nature of an individual's emotional response. He suggests that chronic mourning is frequently predicted by a prolonged period in the shock and numbing phase: the strong, overt expression of affect among chronic mourners is largely disconnected from the situation that elicited it. In other words, intense feelings may be misplaced onto other less important matters, thereby distracting attention from the mourning process. According to Bowlby, unresolved mourning is characterized by the attributes of his second phase of grief – anxiety, searching, and longing – rather than the movement through despair into a measure of acceptance. In comparing unresolved grief to normal grief, Bowlby stated that in normal grief, "Instead of unfocused anxiety, agitation, and despair, there is sadness and longing, combined perhaps with fond memories which, although sad, are not the less intensely pleasurable."

Many authors have warned against overzealous application of time frames in determining whether grief is complicated. Even when mourners express the desire for less intense or a shorter duration of symptoms, it is wise to educate them regarding the variable length of time required for grief to resolve. At the same time it is important not to minimize the unwanted disruption of grief, and not to overlook the possibilities of co-existing clinical disorders.[37]

Functional Impairment

The degree of functional impairment in work and relationships is another important variable used to distinguish complicated mourning from normal bereavement. Although most bereavements do not result in major or prolonged disruptions in functioning, Beverly Raphael concluded from an extensive review of the literature that as many as one-third of bereaved individuals suffer a "morbid outcome or pathological pattern of grief" intense enough to require professional help.[38]

Therese Rando highlights the importance of the client's own evaluation of how well he or she is coping with the death in general, and then specifically in terms of relationships, work, and other responsibilities.[37] Further, clinicians need to help mourners identify the specific challenges they face and determine how well mourners are coping with these challenges. The section on risk analysis below outlines a systematic approach to assessing bereavement burdens and personal impediments to coping, which disrupt functioning.

Symptoms of Complicated Grief

Recent efforts to differentiate complicated and uncomplicated grief have focused on identifying specific grief symptoms that can predict negative bereavement outcomes such as depression, anxiety disorders, and long-term functional impairment. A commonly used research instrument of grief resolution is the Texas Revised Inventory for Grief (TRIG). The TRIG contains an index of grief resolution that includes three statements to test a person's sense of his or her own adjustment: "I feel I have grieved for the person who died," "I feel I have adjusted well to the loss," and "Now I can talk about the person without discomfort."[39]

Using the Grief Resolution Index of the TRIG, Jacquelyn Summers and her colleagues examined AIDS-related grief resolution and psychiatric morbidity in a sample of 286 HIV-positive and HIV-negative gay men between 1989 and 1993.[39] They found that 60 percent of the men reported a loss within the previous twelve months. Eighteen percent of the bereaved men met criteria for unresolved grief. While men with unresolved (complicated) grief were no different from other subjects in terms of lifetime psychiatric disorders, they had an elevated prevalence of current major depression and panic disorder compared to men with uncomplicated grief.

Holly Prigerson and her associates developed an inventory of complicated grief that has been shown to reliably measure maladaptive symptoms of loss.[40] In general Prigerson found that the elements of shock, functionally debilitating intrusive thoughts about the deceased, and resentment because the spouse died, best differentiate persons with complicated grief from those with uncomplicated grief.

Mardi Horowitz, the originator of the concept of the stress response syndrome, proposed the establishment of a diagnostic category of "pathological grief."[41] In this formulation, pathological grief encompasses three categories of symptom-related features: intrusion, denial, and failure to adapt. Intrusions include recurring, unbidden, and uncontrollable conscious experiences, such as haunting thoughts and hard-to-dispel images: memories, images, dreams, and most especially, nightmares. Pangs of fear, sorrow, rage, shame, and guilt may emerge related to the constant feeling of loss of control. Denial (maladaptive avoidance) includes evasion of situations, thoughts, or memories of the deceased. It manifests in psychological numbing and in the diminished ability to make decisions and solve problems. Failure to adapt includes problems working, functioning at home, and forming relationships. (See Table 1: Diagnostic Criteria for Pathological Grief).[41]

In summary, the Integrative Model of AIDS Bereavement defines complicated grief as a disruption in the course of grief as characterized by an atypical intensity (overly numbed or overly intrusive) or duration (absent or chronic) of grief symptoms (shock, numbness, yearning, searching, disorganization, despair), which leads to an unacceptable duration of functional impairment in critical areas of work and relations. In making a diagnosis of complicated grief, clinicians must take into consideration both the mourner's subjective evaluation of his or her progress and the more objective manifestations of complications. Once the clinician ascertains the presence of complicated grief, he or she then moves on to determine whether the mourner also suffers from a co-morbid clinical disorder.

Distinguishing Grief from Mental Disorders

While grief reactions – both complicated and uncomplicated – share symptoms with a variety of mental disorders (for example, affective disorders, post-traumatic stress disorder, and other anxiety disorders), several features distinguish these phenomena. First, grief always exists within a context of loss and is considered both normative and appropriate to this situation. Second, the distinct symptom constellations discussed in the previous section have been reliably used to diagnose complicated grief and differentiate it from other clinical disorders.

When assessing mourners for the presence of complicated grief, it is important to keep in mind that grief reactions may co-exist with psychiatric disorders, a situation known as *co-morbidity.* In order to properly address the needs of mourners, clinicians must determine whether mourners are experiencing complicated grief with or without a co-morbid psychiatric disorder. The two clinical disorders that most commonly co-exist with bereavement are depression and anxiety disorders. Since these conditions also present the greatest challenge in terms of differentiating them from complicated and uncomplicated grief, they receive primary focus in the following discussion.

Depression

While there is a great deal of agreement in the research literature regarding the co-existence of depression and grief, it is difficult to make clear and definitive statements about the prevalence of co-morbidity. The prevalence of depression among mourners ranges in the literature from 30 percent to 80 percent. While most of the research

Table 1. Diagnostic Criteria for Pathological Grief

Reprinted with permission from: Horowitz M, Bonanno G, Holen A. Pathological grief: Diagnosis and explanation. Psychosomatic Medicine. *1993; 55(3): 260-273.*

CRITERIA DESCRIPTION

A. Stressor
   1. Loss of significant other.

B. Intrusion
   1. Occurrence of distressing, intrusive images, ideas, memories, recurrent dreams, or nightmares; the mind is flooded with emotions without a sense of reduction in intensity.
   2. Illusions or pseudo-hallucinations; the mind is "haunted" by a sense of presence of the deceased without a sense of reduction in intensity.

C. Denial
   1. Maladaptive reduction in or avoidance of contemplation in thought, communication, or actions of some important topics related to the loss.
   2. Having an implicit relationship for more than six months with the deceased as if alive; keeping the belongings of the deceased exactly or completely as before.

D. Failure to adapt
   1. Inability to resume work or responsibilities at home beyond one month after the loss.
   2. Barriers to forming new relationships beyond thirteen months after the loss.
   3. Exhaustion, excessive fatigue, or somatic symptoms, having a direct temporal relation to the loss event and persisting beyond one month after the loss.

General rule for the diagnosis of pathological grief: the person must meet criterion A, and must display at least one manifestation within all of the classes B through D. It also is possible to diagnose pathological grief if only one of the criteria from B through D is present to a highly maladaptive degree.

on co-morbidity has studied elderly women, several recent studies have focused on AIDS mourners. Folkman and her colleagues reported that 78 percent of the gay male mourners in their HIV-specific study scored in the depressed range on the Centers for Epidemiology Scale one month after experiencing loss.[27] At the seven-month mark, 53 percent of mourners continued to score in the depressed range.

Although other AIDS bereavement researchers have found somewhat different prevalence rates,[28] the high rate of co-existing depression and grief among AIDS mourners is undeniable. In a rare study that included a demographically mixed sample, Kathleen Sikkema found that depression, traumatic stress, and grief levels were very high among all groups she studied, including African American men and women, as well as gay and bisexual men.[42]

Recent developments in bereavement research have demonstrated empirically the ability to differentiate bereavement depression from other grief reactions. In their investigations of elderly bereaved spouses, Prigerson and her colleagues were able to distinguish grief reactions from bereavement-related depression.[25] They found that seven symptoms comprise a grief reaction: searching, yearning, being preoccupied with thoughts of the deceased, crying, not believing the death had occurred, feeling stunned by the death, and not accepting the death. These symptoms were distinct from the symptoms that comprise bereavement-related depression: hypochondriasis, apathy, insomnia, anxiety, suicidal ideation, guilt, loneliness, depressed mood, psychomotor retardation, hostility, and reduced self-esteem. These grief symptoms were also clearly distinguishable from general anxiety symptoms. Prigerson's demonstration that grief reactions can be differentiated from other psychiatric disorders is central to the organizational scheme presented in this monograph which acknowledges the role of mental disorders in further complicating grief.

Clinicians need to be alert to the possibility of bereavement-related depression throughout the bereavement process, starting in the caregiving stage, continuing through the earliest days of grief, and for several years after. High levels of depressive symptoms found in gay male caregivers prior to a loved one's death and regardless of the HIV status of the caregiver suggest the importance of clinical evaluation and care for caregivers.[27,43]

Finally, several conclusions drawn from the clinical management of depression in general bereavement may be applied to HIV bereavement as well. First, full depressive episodes are common throughout the first year after the death of a spouse. Second, depressive episodes may occur not only in the early months of bereavement, but also later in bereavement. Third, contrary to clinical lore, depressive symptoms early in the mourning process should not be seen as a normal and healthy response to loss, and these symptoms should receive attention sooner rather than later.[44]

Anxiety Disorders

While anxiety is an expected and normal response to loss, anxiety disorders may require psychotherapeutic or pharmacological intervention. Anxiety reactions are often overlooked and may be overshadowed by depressive reactions.[37] Studies have found that both panic disorders – with and without agoraphobia – and generalized anxiety disorders may be associated with bereavement,[44] as may the onset or exacerbation of obsessive-compulsive symptoms. While it is not unusual for there to be anxious avoidance of situations that remind mourners of their losses, when these behaviors significantly interfere with social or occupational functioning, clinicians should consider whether these reactions are evidence of anxiety disorders.[37]

PTSD represents the configuration of symptoms following exposure to an extreme traumatic stressor, that is, the direct experience of an event involving actual or threatened death, or serious injury to oneself or others. This may include witnessing an event that involves death, injury, or a threat to another person; or learning about an unexpected death. To merit a diagnosis, a person's response must involve intense fear, helplessness, or horror. Characteristic symptoms include persistent re-experiencing of the traumatic event, persistent avoidance of stimuli associated with the trauma, and numbing of general responsiveness. Finally, people with PTSD may also suffer from persistent symptoms of increased arousal such as irritability, hypervigilance, and an exaggerated startle response. Distinguishing PTSD from complicated grief is particularly challenging.

Given the overlap of certain symptoms between complicated grief and PTSD – that is, preoccupation with trauma, numbing, intrusive thoughts, and avoidance of reminders – researchers are currently debating whether complicated grief is best classified as a subtype of PTSD. This argument has been fueled by recent changes in the diagnostic criteria of PTSD, which no longer requires that a precipitating event be "beyond the range of usual experience." However, Horowitz points out there are still significant differences between the two. In his words, "Individuals suffering from PTSD may feel out of control because they cannot avoid images that repeat traumatic perceptions: these represent a kind of hypermnesia or an excessive activity of memory." Similar intrusion may occur in what he terms "pathological grief" response (as shown in Table 1: Diagnostic Criteria for Pathological Grief). Yet a considerable portion of the intrusions may arise in relation to memories or images that serve as essentially positive and temporarily comforting portrayals of the deceased still alive.[41]

Using data from the Stanford HIV Caregiving and Bereavement Study, Joel Friedman found that while most AIDS mourners experienced some of the symptoms of PTSD, including intrusive thinking and affective numbing, few met the complete criteria for a diagnosis of PTSD.[28] An important diagnostic distinction regards the nature of intrusive images and whether these images directly relate to the traumatic situation. Furthermore, conceptualizing complicated grief as a subset of PTSD obscures aspects of complicated grief such as whether a person is adequately managing the stages and tasks of grief. Under the Integrative Model presented in this monograph, therefore, clients may meet criteria for either or both complicated grief and PTSD. (For an example of a differential diagnosis of complicated grief and PTSD, see the case of Paul presented in Chapter 3.)

Risk Factors for AIDS Bereavement Distress

Most bereaved individuals are able to manage the burdens of grief, relying on their own personal resources, without major or prolonged disruptions in their daily functioning. The empirical literature concludes that most bereaved people – both traditional and AIDS bereaved – demonstrate little psychological or physical impairment twelve to eighteen months after a loss.[18,27,28] On the other hand, a sizable minority – an estimated one-third – of mourners experience bereavement distress great enough to require some level of professional assistance.[38] Why are some people able to manage the stress of losing a loved one while others are not? Researchers and clinicians have attempted to identify factors that predict various forms of bereavement distress. The term *risk factors* is commonly used to indicate characteristics that either increase a person's vulnerability to a loss experience or slow adjustment and recovery.[1] In contrast, *resilience* refers to a person's ability to adapt to loss and its associated strains with minimal psychological distress and psychosocial impairment.

It is important to note several cautions before applying empirical findings related to bereavement risk and resilience to clinical practice. First, while bereavement studies ideally include a non-bereaved comparison group, not all studies have followed this procedure. Second, most of the empirical studies follow the bereaved for relatively short durations of time: several weeks or months, sometimes one year, with only a few studies following the bereaved for up to two years. Third, many of these factors have been studied primarily within the context of conjugal bereavement and most with elderly or at least middle-aged women, thereby limiting their generalizability to the larger bereavement population and particularly to the AIDS bereaved. Finally, different methodologies across studies – different time frames, different measures, different definitions – add further complexity to an interpretation and integration of the risk factor literature.[1]

The risk factors discussed in the following sections have either an empirical basis or a strong theoretical rationale for the prediction of negative AIDS bereavement outcomes. In addition to actual predictors of poor bereavement outcome, the list includes some factors that have been shown to simply be associated with poor bereavement outcome; this allows a broader conceptualization of the combination of factors that place a person at risk. Being as inclusive as this, even when the research is equivocal, increases the selection of mourners at some level of risk. In other words, it allows clinicians to identify the greatest number of people possibly in need of some form of assistance. Once such clients have been identified, appropriate treatment requires more careful evaluation to determine the type of assistance that is necessary.

Risk Analysis in the Integrative Model for AIDS Bereavement

Risk analysis in the Integrative Model for AIDS Bereavement divides risk factors into two categories: *bereavement burdens* and *personal impediments to coping.* (See Table 2: Risk Factors for AIDS Bereavement Distress for a listing of all of these factors.) The theoretical and empirical work of Susan Folkman suggests the value of taking both of these categories into consideration when determining an individual mourner's risk. Folkman conceptualizes bereavement burden as being comprised of the potential stressors or demands placed on the mourner. Her work also suggests the importance of assessing not only the bereavement demands a client faces but also his or her personal resources to cope with these demands;[27] in this context, impediments to coping reflect characteristics or ongoing

Table 2. Risk Factors for AIDS Bereavement Distress

BEREAVEMENT BURDENS

1. Being HIV-infected.
2. Being a caregiver, primary partner or spouse, or parent.
3. Perceiving interpersonal conflict or a lack of social support.
4. Experiencing an accumulation of stressors (including multiple losses).
5. Being young.
6. Experiencing difficulty resolving a relationship with the deceased, (including an unexpected death, or an ambivalent or especially close relationship with the deceased).

PERSONAL IMPEDIMENTS TO COPING

1. Tendency to engage in ineffective and avoidance coping.
2. Tendency to over-engage in self-focused attention (including ruminative coping).
3. Tendency to experience guilt and lowered self-esteem (including internalized homophobia).
4. Tendency toward negative thinking (including a pessimistic outlook).
5. Current substance abuse or dependency.

problems that interfere with a person's ability to accurately appraise and cope with bereavement stress.

In interpreting the diagnostic value of any of these risk factors, it is important to note that single factors typically do not predict specific negative bereavement outcomes. Concern should be heightened by both the magnitude of each risk factor and the number of risk factors identified. For example, the clinical response would be different for a client whose support network is merely being taxed compared to the client who, after the loss of a partner, is left totally isolated. It is also important to understand how risk factors relate to each other. This is especially true in terms of the overall relationship between personal impediments to coping and bereavement burdens. For example, is a person's pessimistic style (an impediment to coping) blocking him or her from making new friends and having satisfying social relationships (a bereavement burden relating to the lack of social support)? The following review of risk factors – first bereavement burdens and then personal impediments to coping – aims to assist clinicians in identifying those AIDS mourners who are most at risk for complicated grief or psychiatric disorders.

Bereavement Burdens

Burden 1: Being HIV-Infected

Clearly, being HIV-infected places an extra burden on anyone, including those who mourn. It is not uncommon to hear a seropositive mourner ask with fear and anguish, "Who will be there to take care of *me*?" Of course, the state of a seropositive person's health plays a role in the magnitude of this burden, and the level of perceived threat from HIV infection may be somewhat diminished in light of the success of new medical treatments: optimism may diminish stress. On the other hand, treatment failure may once again heighten bereavement distress.

Throughout the epidemic, research findings have been mixed relative to the predictive value of seropositivity on bereavement distress. Some studies have found a predictive relationship,[45] others have not.[39,43] More recently, Folkman found that HIV status predicted depressive mood in bereaved caregivers, but the effect she found was relatively small.[27] Specifically, during the months immediately after the death of their partners, seropositive caregivers were no more depressed than their uninfected counterparts: all bereaved caregivers were significantly depressed during this period. However, seven months after the death of a partner, the two groups had diverged: the depressive mood of uninfected caregivers tended to diminish, whereas it tended to remain high among seropositive caregivers.

Burden 2: Being a Caregiver, Spouse, Primary Partner, or Parent

The psychological stress of caregiving is well-documented. A review of the empirical literature shows that caregivers experience high levels of perceived burden and stress, along with disrupted family life, financial burdens, and psychological symptoms including depression, sleep problems, severe fatigue, anxiety, and feelings of hopelessness about the future.[46] Furthermore, in a finding that has direct relevance for many HIV caregivers, caregivers to family members with a progressive dementia are likely to be highly distressed as death represents not only a loss, but also a relief.[47] In studying gay male partners who served as primary caregivers, Folkman found that despite sociodemographic differences, gay caregivers and traditional family caregivers had comparable severity, duration, and variability of bereavement-related depressive mood.[27]

While AIDS caregiving responsibilities often fall to primary partners, a variety of caregiving arrangements include parents, friends, and community volunteers. Research with gay men suggests that caregivers, both the partners and mothers of HIV-infected people, are at increased risk for psychological distress.[45] Sarah Erickson found that gay male caregivers had high levels of depressive symptoms, regardless of their own HIV or health status. These results suggest that the demands of the caregiving role supersede any palliative or deleterious effect of personal health or multiple loss.[43]

Although there is little empirical data, social and clinical observation suggests added strain on parents who mourn a loss to HIV disease, and it is notable that parental mourning is, in itself, a predictor for complicated grief. Further, parents of both gay men and injection drug users may be estranged from their children, and this estrangement may lead to an exacerbation of guilt and remorse after the death of the child. In addition, parents of young HIV-infected children are likely to be infected themselves. In fact, many have transmitted HIV to their children perinatally, a situation that may represent the most difficult and high-risk bereavement, replete with self-blame, "survivor guilt," and increased or renewed drug use among injection drug users.

For many parents of people who have died from AIDS, grief is exacerbated by the perceived need to maintain secrecy and by shame and guilt.[37] This guilt and shame, or fear that others will negatively judge them, may prevent mourners from seeking support from community resources. Adult seropositive children often return home during the terminal phase of the illness, a reverse migration from large urban areas to smaller rural or suburban areas where HIV is less prevalent. Culture shock for the child combined with lack of support for both the parent and child may lead to conflict before the death and remorse on the part of the parental mourner afterwards.[37]

Burden 3: Perceiving Conflict or a Lack of Social Support

Perhaps the area of greatest agreement between the clinical and research literature on predicting bereavement outcomes regards the role of perceived social support in mediating psychological health. The accumulated research suggests that the perception of social support is more important than any quantitative measure of support.[48] It has found a connection between a perceived lack of social support and poor bereavement outcomes as measured by poor health in the first year of bereavement,[38,49,50] heightened distress two years after the loss,[51] and an increased use of anti-anxiety medications.[48,52] In fact, one study found that the single best predictor of heightened distress one month following loss is a lack of contact with friends who had distanced themselves during a lengthy illness.[53]

Certain subjective qualities of social support have been associated with psychological well-being and distress in gay male caregivers of loved ones with HIV disease.[43] Specifically, individuals who felt overall satisfaction with their social networks had lower levels of distress. Affirmation – approval of one's beliefs, feelings, and decisions by important others – has also been found to be helpful to mourners.[54,55]

Conflict and friction within the social network may have a negative impact on emotional well-being. Erickson found that the amount of friction in a gay male caregiver's network, the frequency of unpleasant encounters, and social isolation were the most consistent and strongly related support measures associated with depression. Parents and other relatives may find themselves in conflict with partners and "chosen family" of their ill or deceased adult children. These two groups may find themselves in a battle for loyalty, attention, and the right to care for their loved one. This conflict may persist after the death in arenas such as post-death rituals and estate settlement and may add bereavement burden to these mourners.[37]

Burden 4: Experiencing an Accumulation of Stressors

Bereavement distress has been associated with the sheer number of stressors that arise during the mourning process.[38] These additional stressors may include unemployment, relationship breakup, the loss of physical health, and daily hassles. Another stressor, financial hardship, may also lead to lowered morale, decreased affiliation and social participation, increased loneliness and anxiety, poor adjustment, and negative health outcomes among bereaved individuals.[56-58]

Researchers have hypothesized that the accumulation of loss is a stressor that must play a role in bereavement distress. The role of multiple loss in predicting bereavement distress, however, is complicated and still not clearly understood. Fortunately, given the dramatic reductions in HIV-related deaths due to new medical treatments, such clustering of deaths may become less common. On the other hand, it is clear that many AIDS mourners will continue to suffer from the experience of multiple losses for many years to come. To add to the concrete losses due to death and of functioning due to poor physical health, many mourners suffer from a variety of symbolic losses – for example, the loss of sexual freedom or the loss of a sense of community – due to the epidemic.

There are many clinical examples of clients who have come to therapy overwhelmed by the accumulation of losses due to AIDS deaths and the devastation of core support systems due to the disease. Empirical research, however, has not found a clear relationship between multiple bereavement and specific forms of bereavement distress. Studies conducted early in the epidemic suggested that the cumulative effects of multiple deaths made individuals more vulnerable to psychological distress.[59] Later studies, however, have not supported this earlier observation.[45] Richard Neugebauer and his colleagues found that neither the overall level of depressive symptoms, the presence of specific symptom clusters, nor the presence of a diagnosed depressive disorder was related to the number of AIDS deaths reported by a subject.[60] While the experience of multiple deaths does not seem to have a direct effect on bereavement distress, multiple deaths may add to bereavement burden if they have a significant impact on the amount and quality of social support and if they are accompanied by other risk factors such as seropositivity.

Burden 5: Being Young

As the demographics of the epidemic in the United States change, more and more young people are exposed to the HIV-related death of a parent, sibling, or friend. Many of the children coping with the death of a parent are also poor and have had a parent with substance abuse problems. Obviously, those children who find themselves homeless after the death of a parent represent a high-risk for a variety of negative bereavement outcomes. While children have not been extensively studied, the bereavement literature offers some insight into the risks for children surviving an HIV-related death.

Although there is general agreement that the death of a parent is a stressful experience for school-aged children,[61] and some researchers have found that such losses can lead to depression or behavior problems among these children, such findings have not been universal. Additional factors, including the way the surviving parent responds to the child, the availability of social support, and life circumstances such as a troubled parental remarriage, seem to make a difference in whether children develop emotional problems.[62] One study found that the children with the highest level of bereavement distress – including disturbed behavior – were those who had the poorest peer support and lowest self-esteem and who felt that they had the least control.[61]

Burden 6: Difficulty Resolving a Relationship with the Deceased

A number of prospective research studies and clinical commentaries have suggested that the nature of the relationship between the mourner and the deceased is a factor in determining the course of mourning.[63,64] Psychoanalyst Simon Rubin suggests that:

> *The dynamic relationship of the bereaved to the memories and associations of the deceased determine resolution [of grief]. . . . Ambivalent or conflictual relationships with the deceased make more difficult accepting the reality of death, reducing yearning for reuniting, and re-establishing relationships with others.*[65]

On the other hand, Camille Wortman suggests that another group at risk for complicated grief are those who mourn the loss of an extremely good relationship, the absence of which shatters their view of the world as controllable, predictable, and safe.[18]

The empirical evidence regarding the impact of sudden, unexpected, and untimely deaths is also inconsistent. Some studies have found that unexpectedness of the loss has a negative impact on health outcomes; others, primarily ones in which subjects were elderly, did not reach this conclusion. One study found that the combination of unexpected loss plus the subject's belief that he or she had little control over what happens was a significant risk factor for both somatic and depressive complaints. For such individuals, an unexpected death may strengthen this sense of powerlessness and lead to withdrawal, resignation, and minimal efforts to recover from grief.[1]

Robert Weiss and T. Anne Richards evaluated narratives from gay caregivers in Susan Folkman's study to determine whether attachment theory could predict bereavement outcomes.[66] They hypothesized that since "unforewarned loss made for difficulties in recovery . . . [it] would be experienced as inexplicable abandonment and would therefore give rise to a search for fault in the attachment figure and the self and to wariness regarding new relationships of attachment." The researchers found that the ability of the caregiver to anticipate a partner's death and the caregiver's lack of ambivalence toward the deceased were positively correlated with personal adjustment. These findings again suggest that a broad approach to risk factor assessment is necessary, one that is multifactorial in nature.

Personal Impediments to Coping

Impediment 1: Ineffective and Avoidance Coping

Using ineffective methods to cope with bereavement-related problems may relate to the nature of the current stressor or to a more generalized impediment in coping abilities. Many mourners fall back on old patterns such as overeating, substance use, or inappropriate sexual behavior to try to avoid the pain of grief. For example, substance dependence may be understood as a maladaptive avoidance coping behavior when it is used in lieu of more productive problem-solving and emotion-focused strategies. In this way, it may interfere with adequate mourning and may put the mourner at risk for negative physical and psychological outcomes.

Many studies of the effect of coping on psychological distress have shown that avoidance and denial, as forms of emotion-focused coping, are associated with depressed mood[67,68] and problem-focused coping is associated with reduced distress.[69,70] These findings have been replicated with studies of gay men coping with HIV disease.[71,72]

Susan Folkman identified factors that distinguished those gay mourners whose depression decreased over time from those whose depression showed little change or increased.[27] She found that finding meaning in caregiving had a positive effect on recovery, while distancing and self-blame coping strategies predicted undiminished depressed mood. Those who fared better were future-oriented, had positive goals for themselves, and experienced positive emotions upon achieving these goals. The depressed men were more likely to deny a partner's death and were more focused on wishful thinking about recapturing aspects of the relationship with the partner.

Impediment 2: Self-Focused Attention and Ruminative Coping

Contrary to much clinical lore, the tendency to spend an inordinate amount of time in self-reflection and being self-focused is more detrimental than helpful. Self-focused attention has been defined as the disposition to analyze one's personality and internal states regardless of mood.[73] This tendency to dwell on one's inner life has been associated with higher prevalence of negative self-evaluation and depression.[74] In several laboratory studies, depressed subjects placed in situations in which they were required to maintain their attention on inner emotional states, experienced an increase in negative affect, while subjects who were encouraged to focus away from the self – in other words distraction – experienced a reduction in negative mood. Other studies have found that depressed individuals made to focus on themselves have more pessimistic expectancies of future events and remember more negative events from the past.[75]

Susan Nolen-Hoeksema and her colleagues identified a form of self-focus which they call "ruminative coping."[76,77] In this state people worry excessively but passively about their depression, its symptoms, the implications of their depression, and the consequences that being depressed has on their lives. While this rumination may appear to be a method to solve problems ("What am I going to do now?"), it is actually associated with greater distress and the ruminative person is less likely to engage in active problem-solving behavior. Hence, bereaved individuals who engage in more analysis of themselves and the meaning of their loss show more persistent depression and absence of positive states of mind after their loss. In a large cancer-based caregiving and bereavement study, Nolen-Hoeksema demonstrated that people who are overly focused on their emotions are at risk for more severe and lengthy periods of distress.[55]

In a re-examination of narratives generated in Folkman's study, Nolen-Hoeksema found that bereaved men with more negative ruminative thoughts in free-response interviews showed greater psychological distress on several outcome measures both one month and twelve months after their loss and less increase in positive morale over the twelve-month period.[77] Men who engaged in more analysis of themselves and the meaning of their loss reported greater positive morale one month after their loss but showed persistent depression and absence of positive states of mind over the twelve months following the loss. While the coding of ruminative thinking was done after the fact using written accounts rather than interviews, it appears to demonstrate that self-analysis, when used in excess, can interfere with other forms of positive coping.

Impediment 3: Guilt and Lowered Self-Esteem

For some mourners, guilt may arise in response to their own negative evaluation of their caregiving performance; for others, it may be the result of long-standing psychological problems. Some gay and bisexual mourners may experience lower self-esteem related to internalized homophobia: the incorporation of negative attitudes and beliefs about homosexuality into one's self-image and gay or lesbian identity.[78]

Guilt may arise when caregivers believe that they were not able or willing to provide the care that their loved one needed when he or she was alive. Families who kept the illness of a loved one secret or for whom the fear of contagion prompted exaggerated precautions may find it difficult to forgive themselves.[37] At times, such self-reproach may be warranted, as in the case of families who have abandoned their relatives; at other times, the self-reproach is overly harsh and unrealistic. In either case, it may complicate bereavement.

Finally, even those gay men who have lived for years feeling good about their sexuality may be revisited by the negative self-images and associated anguish of internalized homophobia when confronted by a stressful event of the magnitude of the loss of a partner. In some ways, the unhappiness associated with disease and death may seem to validate early negative predictions given about being gay. In a study of gay men where bereavement was not the focus, greater internalized homophobia predicted greater psychological distress two years after baseline.[79] This finding was especially strong for seropositive men, but disease progression was not associated with internalized homophobia, coping, or psychological distress. However, research on bereaved gay men has not clearly documented the prevalence of any associated negative effects of internalized homophobia. In fact, most research has shown gay men to be highly resilient in the face of the stresses presented by HIV disease.[79] In a study of seropositive gay men (not necessarily mourners), few respondents had high levels of internalized homophobia, but for those who did, it was correlated with psychological distress.

Impediment 4: Negative Thinking

In general, people with an optimistic appraisal style demonstrate greater emotional well-being than those who are more pessimistic.[80,81] In a caregiver study, Nolen-Hoeksema found that, although pessimism was correlated with depression in family members of the terminally ill, it did not remain a significant predictor when social support and coping skills were taken into account.[82] She speculated that pessimism about the future is realistic for these people and that adaptive coping and available social support were associated with lower depression. While this may be true, it is important to note that optimism is correlated with social support. Perhaps optimists find it easier to reach out for help, or people are more disposed to helping individuals who are more optimistic. In addition, optimists report using more distraction and problem-solving coping strategies and less rumination and avoidance.

Sarah Erickson found that gay male caregivers who had greater levels of both general optimism and HIV-related optimism (beliefs that one could cope well with HIV disease, for example) reported less distress.[43] Not surprisingly, men who were generally optimistic were also optimistic regarding the threat of HIV, and this was true regardless of serostatus. This type of investigation has not been conducted among mourners, so one can only speculate that optimism prior to the loss would continue at some level, perhaps attenuated, and therefore predict less distress after the loss.

Impediment 5: Current Substance Abuse or Dependency

The relationship between substance abuse and HIV-related bereavement is a complex one. Substance abuse can be both a risk factor for bereavement distress and a negative outcome of painful bereavement. A sizable and growing proportion of people with HIV disease have been infected as a result of unsafe injection drug use, and clinical observation suggests that those mourning the loss of these individuals are more likely to have a current or past history of substance abuse, be at increased risk of psychological distress, and be HIV-infected themselves. They are also more likely to be isolated, stigmatized, and experience financial difficulties.

Research has documented an increased prevalence in prescription and non-prescription drug, alcohol, and tobacco use among mourners.[83] Although some increase in substance use is attributable to new use, much reflects increased use by individuals already using substances. The heavy use of mind-altering substances may interfere with successful bereavement in several ways. Using drugs and alcohol to anesthetize the pain of grief may block, delay, or prolong the mourning process. On the other hand, some mourners actually reduce or stop, at least for a while, their intake of their drug of choice during bereavement. In these cases, the expression of grief may be clouded by alcohol or drug withdrawal symptoms. In both cases, emotional responses that arise may either be related to the experience of loss or be artifacts of intoxication or withdrawal. Several authors have reported research indicating that bereaved alcoholics are at higher risk for suicide, both deliberate and unintentional.[37] Furthermore, increased substance use during bereavement has been documented to be associated with increased behavioral changes that compromise health maintenance or chronic disease management.[83]

AIDS Bereavement Resilience

Both the general and AIDS bereavement literatures are quite clear on one fact: most mourners are able to navigate the course of grief without long-term detrimental effects.[6,27,84] Robert Mcrae and Paul Costa argue that the evidence supports the conclusion that mourners are for the most part "resilient." They hold that after the period of intense grief is over, there is a return to a "baseline" level of well-being comparable to that of non-bereaved individuals.[85] While there is a growing empirical and research literature regarding factors that predict the subset of mourners at risk for heightened bereavement distress, little work has addressed factors that predict those who show resilience in the face of mourning. Nowhere is this resilience to bereavement distress more apparent than in gay men who have weathered the AIDS epidemic.

In a now classic article, John Martin and Laura Dean examined the influence of AIDS-related bereavement on psychological distress of gay men in New York between 1985 and 1991.[45] To their surprise they found that – even in the face of multiple losses – the intensity and duration of bereavement effects diminished over time rather than resulting in a cumulative negative effect. This led them to speculate that gay men were adapting to the epidemic: over time, these men learned to cope better with the epidemic's stresses.

Susan Folkman's research offers some ideas about what is required to be resilient in the face of AIDS bereavement. She found that bereaved individuals who were able to react to ongoing stresses by systematically appraising the situation, setting realistic goals for reducing the stress, and taking positive action during the caregiving process fared better up to twelve months after their loss. Furthermore, caregivers who evaluated events relatively more positively were able to formulate realistic goals and plans.[27,72]

The issue of risk and resilience is complex, and findings about these concepts are at times equivocal. While systematic research can provide some guidance and a check on clinical bias, it does not provide an unambiguous pathway to understanding who will and who will not grieve well. Clinicians seeking to help AIDS mourners can be guided by the multifactorial assessment of risk factors provided above. At the same time, clinicians must not use these risk factors in a cookbook fashion. There are many subtleties to AIDS-related grief work – and grief work in general. As Shuchter and Zisook admonish: "There are large individual differences among mourners."[86] Individualized assessment of risk and resilience must combine objective measures with clinical judgment to derive the most accurate picture of current functioning as well as to predict future adjustment.

Conclusion: Assessing AIDS Bereavement Distress

The best way to understand the variance in adaptation to an AIDS bereavement is to listen carefully to mourners themselves. It is important to understand each client within the cultural, historical, and personal context of his or her life. What special meaning does the client give each loss? What meaning does he or she give to the aggregate experience of facing the AIDS epidemic? What is the client's perception of how well he or she is doing?

Grounded in humility in the face of uncertainty and guided by the Integrative Model, clinicians are prepared to assess the type and level of bereavement distress AIDS mourners exhibit:

- By applying the criteria for distinguishing complicated from uncomplicated grief, the clinician is able to determine whether the client is adequately moving through the course of grieving.
- By applying standard diagnostic procedures (DSM-IV), the clinician is able to identify the presence of co-morbid clinical disorders.
- By using the catalog of AIDS Bereavement Risk Factors, the clinician is able to identify mourners at risk for future complications or exacerbation of current bereavement distress and also to identify areas of strength and resilience.

Based on this assessment, the clinician can determine the type and level of AIDS bereavement distress. Chapter Three describes the range of activities and interventions that may be applied based on this differential assessment of AIDS bereavement distress.

3

Helping the AIDS Mourner

WHILE in most cases of AIDS bereavement, individuals are able to manage the emotional and physical impact of grief with the support of their friends, family, and community, clinicians may be called upon to assist people at every level of bereavement distress. Following a careful assessment of the type and level of bereavement distress, clinicians can construct a treatment plan that may include a combination of individual, small group, and community-wide activities. (See Table 3: Level of Bereavement Distress and Potential Interventions for an outline of the Integrative Model.)

Effective bereavement interventions range from educational activities to psychotherapy. This chapter describes these activities and a method for matching activities and mourners. Finally, it proposes a psychotherapeutic approach – Integrative AIDS Bereavement Therapy – that combines aspects of psychodynamic and cognitive behavioral therapy and is enhanced by recent developments specifically designed to assist AIDS mourners in reducing their risk for complicated grief.

Table 3. Level of Bereavment Distress and Potential Interventions

Level of Distress	Bereavement Interventions			
One: Uncomplicated Mourning without Risk Factors	AIDS Bereavement Education and Support			
Two: Uncomplicated Mourning with Risk Factors	AIDS Bereavement Education and Support	Bereavement Risk Reduction Counseling		
Three: Complicated Mourning without Clinical Disorder	AIDS Bereavement Education and Support	Bereavement Risk Reduction Counseling	Grief-Related Psychotherapy	
Four: Complicated Mourning with Clinical Disorder	AIDS Bereavement Education and Support	Bereavement Risk Reduction Counseling	Grief-Related Psychotherapy	Psychiatric Evaluation and Treatment

Communities vary in terms of the services available for AIDS mourners. To some degree, the extent of services is consistent with the magnitude of the problem. That is, those communities hardest hit by the epidemic, especially those with large populations of middle-class gay men, have established the most extensive support systems. The first step for clinicians is to determine the types of services available in their communities. Once this resource map is constructed, clinicians can match mourners to appropriate bereavement interventions based on the individualized assessment described in Chapter Two. While a discussion of community-wide health planning is outside the scope of this monograph, it is important to note that the array of AIDS bereavement interventions described here can be useful in designing a community-wide response to this problem.

Educational and Support Approaches

AIDS bereavement education and support may take a variety of forms and cover a range of topics. Through written material, conversations with friends, or formal discussions with helping professionals, AIDS mourners learn about the universal nature of bereavement and the unique aspects of AIDS bereavement, the signs of bereavement distress, the definitions of effective coping strategies, and ways to find bereavement activities and services in their community. Whether one-on-one or within groups, bereavement education and support can go a long way toward assisting mourners in coping with their grief and preventing bereavement-related problems.

In the early stages of grief, people often say that they are unprepared for the intensity of their feelings and the level of disruption these feelings cause, and they are relieved to hear that such experiences are normal. Throughout the course of AIDS grief, mourners are assisted by knowledge and encouragement regarding what to expect of the grief process. Bereavement education is helpful to mourners at all levels of bereavement distress and may be delivered in a variety of venues and through a variety of sources such as physicians or other medical personnel, mental health providers, clergy or spiritual leaders, or friends and family members.

Community-Level Education and Support

Broad-based AIDS education may help to mediate the stigma associated with HIV disease and may provide an opportunity for healing on the largest scale. Sympathetic films and television programs have helped to change general attitudes toward people with HIV and may assist distressed mourners who may be reluctant to reach out for help. Community-wide rituals such as memorial services and candlelight parades may alleviate the sense that those who have died have been devalued and forgotten. Participating in ceremonies such as the unfolding of the AIDS Memorial Quilt may provide an opportunity to mourn with others. Elizabeth Taylor's description of her reaction to the Quilt offers a good example of the power of community-wide rituals.

> *The Quilt gives us our most direct feelings back; our feelings of belonging, our sense of precariousness of life, why it is worth clinging to, how it can be lived, how tragically it can be lost, how beautifully, after all, it can be relinquished, and how vibrantly it can be remembered.*[87]

Cleve Jones, in describing his decision to create the Quilt, states:

We wanted to illustrate the enormity of the AIDS crisis by revealing something of the lives behind the statistics, to provide evidence of the calamity that we saw unfolding. We wanted to reach out to all the different kinds of people whose lives had been invaded by AIDS so that they could be strengthened in their personal struggles. And we wanted to give the world a powerful symbol of compassion and unity, an example of how we expected people everywhere to respond to this terrible challenge.[88]

Whether through media, community-wide rituals and celebrations, or stated public policies, communities can make a positive difference in the lives of AIDS mourners by establishing a context of tolerance and compassion for all people affected by HIV disease. Community-wide messages that emphasize the universality of pain and suffering associated with all chronic and life-threatening illnesses help destigmatize HIV disease. At the same time messages that identify the unique challenges of HIV validate the belief that AIDS requires specific efforts tailored to address these challenges.

Education and Support Provided by Helping Professionals

Through the course of HIV disease, most seropositive individuals and those who care for them encounter a wide variety of helping professionals, including medical personnel, social services workers, and religious or spiritual advisors. Sensitivity to bereavement issues on the part of these professionals can assist potential mourners to prepare for a death, help recent mourners cope with the loss, and identify mourners who may need additional help adjusting to the experience.

Clergy

Bereavement education is often provided through spiritual sources such as clergy or religious lay persons. These efforts may help mourners place death within an overall religious or philosophical context, thus reducing their sense of alienation. Secular counselors must be sensitive to religious and cultural differences among mourners and should encourage mourners to find ways to cope with mourning consistent with their own religious, cultural, and personal values. Sympathetic religious personnel can go a long way toward assisting mourners to reconcile religious beliefs with the HIV-associated stigma.

HIV disease poses a dilemma for many religious leaders. While some liberal clergy have been on the forefront of preaching tolerance and love for people with HIV and those who love them, others have used AIDS as a rallying cry for more intolerant religious perspectives. The pain of isolation from one's religious community is poignantly demonstrated by the following excerpts from a letter to the AIDS Quilt newsletter *On Display.*[89]

True Story Three: A Story of Grief and Inspiration

> *My name is Rosetta DuBois-Gadson. I am an ordained minister of the African Methodist Episcopal Church. I am also a mother who has lost a child to AIDS. On May 30, 1994, my son Craig was rushed to Beth Israel Hospital in New York City. When I spoke to him that night on the phone he told me not to worry, that it was just a parasite – cryptosporidium – that he had probably gotten when he was on his last trip to Mexico. . . . It wasn't until July 5th that Craig took my hand and told me that he had something he wanted to tell me himself because we had never kept anything from each other. . . . He told me he was positive. He discovered it in 1990 when he applied for insurance, but he told no one. I grieved then and I grieve now for the isolation my son endured. I needed to know why, WHY couldn't he tell me? So I asked and he answered, "I knew that you, my mother, my best friend, Rosetta, would be there for me, but I didn't know if Reverend Rosetta DuBois-Gadson would be. . . ."*
>
> *AIDS was, and still continues to be, so abhorrent to many church leaders and members that they turn their backs on it. And I just learned that my own son feared that this part of me would do the same! There came a revelation that I can only describe as divine. I was filled with righteous indignation and I could feel the strength building in me. My rage had to be transformed into action. All fear had to leave me because I was being launched into a new ministry that I never would have imagined.*

Craig died two-and-a-half years later.

Rosetta DuBois-Gadson has kept her promise to work actively as a pastor and AIDS educator and is committed to do so until, in her words, "The African American community can show the world that we are not afraid to speak, not afraid to love *all* our children." While inspirational religious leaders like Rosetta DuBois-Gadson are few, a great deal can be done to relieve the suffering of AIDS mourners by clergy less dedicated to AIDS work. Perhaps the most importantly step is for religious workers to bring this issue out in the open and to speak positively about those who suffer from the epidemic.

Medical Providers

Medical personnel, especially those in primary care, are often in a position to provide counsel to caregivers and mourners and must assess whether individuals would benefit from more formal bereavement education, bereavement risk reduction counseling, psychotherapy, or psychopharmacological interventions. George and Adrian Burnell, in *Clinical Management of Bereavement: A Handbook for Health Care Professionals,* suggest that medical personnel need to be aware of common bereavement myths and be able to dispel those that serve as obstacles to healthy grieving.[90] These myths fall into several general categories: that time heals all wounds, that emotions should be avoided or curtailed, that there are strict time parameters for grieving, and that drugs and alcohol can ease the pain of grieving. It is also useful for medical providers to understand and discuss the role of psychopharmacological agents in mourning in a way which neither sends the message that the pain of grief is pathological nor denies medical relief when it is needed and can be effective.

In advising physicians about grief and mourning, Stephen Shuchter and Sidney Zisook warn against counseling patients to "get past their loss" or to "put it behind them."[91] Physicians need to be sensitive to the fact that important connections do not end when a loved one dies. Shuchter and Zisook point out that the death of a loved one is forever, and elements of a survivor's grief will also last forever. Rather than persuading mourners to complete their grieving, Shuchter and Zisook advise medical providers to give mourners permission to maintain some form of ongoing relationship with the deceased. This may include allowing themselves to have conversations with the deceased.

Medical providers may explain that it is common for mourners to identify with the deceased in such a way that they incorporate certain aspects or behaviors of their loved ones. Rather than hurry mourning along, Shuchter and Zisook suggest that, "It is helpful for patients to know that you care, to listen when they feel like talking, to offer the perspective of someone who identifies with the painful and often protracted course of grief, and to be ready to step in when, and if, a major depression or other medical or psychiatric complications develop." This sensitivity may be particularly helpful to persons who mourn an AIDS death and who may be experiencing or expecting rejection from others, especially those they perceive to be in authority.

Finally, given the chronic nature of HIV disease, physicians often develop ongoing relationships not only with the seropositive individual, but also with his or her loved ones. Many people with HIV disease are involved in nontraditional relationships – most notably with gay partners and alternative family members – and for such individuals, the mourning process may be complicated by the lack of validation for the relationships they grieve. A respectful attitude by the physician to these nontraditional caregivers may serve to reinforce and validate the relationships, making the subsequent mourning process a bit easier.

AIDS Bereavement Support Groups

A variety of bereavement support group formats – professional and self-help; time-limited and open-ended – may assist AIDS mourners. While research specific to AIDS bereavement support groups is minimal, considerable data is available suggesting the positive effects of support groups for mourners in reducing the risk to both physical and mental health.[92]

Decisions related to the nature and composition of AIDS bereavement support groups are dictated by a variety of factors including community resources, prevalence of HIV disease within a community, and specific objectives of the group. One question is determining the degree of heterogeneity of mourners to include in the group. AIDS crosses many lines of culture, class, and sexual orientation. While advantages of universality can be engendered in heterogeneous groups, mourning may not be the time to experiment with the tolerance of diversity. Another question is whether the group should be self-help or professionally led. Finally, the duration of the group is important to consider when selecting a support group. Most mourners find that after a brief time, usually eight to twelve weeks, they are ready to cope with their losses supported by people already in their lives. On the other hand, some mourners find themselves without adequate support and may opt for an ongoing group format.

Self-Help Bereavement Support Groups

Self-help groups are characterized by the coming together of participants around a common condition or symptom, situation, heritage, or experience. These groups are self-governing and value self-reliance and accessibility without charge. Leadership in these groups varies; there may be peer facilitators, rotating leadership among participants, or no leaders at all. Many people find attending self-help groups more acceptable than relying on professionals, whom they may view with some suspicion.[92] As is true for groups led by professional leaders, self-help groups provide education and information, personal support, and an opportunity to receive assistance with decision-making and problem-solving. They also provide an opportunity to observe others who are further along in the grief process and who may serve as role models for more newly bereaved individuals.

The procedures and tone of self-help groups tend to be less formal than those of professionally led groups. Members are encouraged to have contact with each other outside of group meetings, and often meetings are held in members' homes rather than in institutional settings. Community organizations typically sponsor these self-help efforts, providing training to leaders or training materials to help guide the groups.

The self-help nature of the group tends to reinforce a nonpathological view of grieving. Given the level of stigmatization associated with HIV disease, having others whose experiences are similar helps to normalize and universalize mourners' grief reactions. Often a strong group cohesion forms and members thrive on a sense of belonging and unconditional acceptance. In some cases this cohesion is fostered by perceptions of "outsider status," with an undercurrent of separation from "those who don't understand us" and a bonding together against a hostile world.

While self-help groups are generally useful, there are some risks associated with this format. Appropriate matching of an individual to the group is extremely important. Care is required in determining whether the philosophy and group process is suitable for the individual. Some groups emphasize expression of intense emotions and may coerce individuals to be more emotionally disclosive than they are comfortable being. Other groups are guided by specific political or philosophical principles and may not be open to individual variation. The absence of professional leadership may also be problematic when individuals with disruptive personalities enter a group and act inappropriately. Therefore, it is important to understand the nature of each group and determine its appropriateness for an individual before recommending it to a client.

Professionally-Led Bereavement Support Groups

Where self-help groups have a cost advantage and run less risk of being stigmatizing, having a professional leader provides an element of quality control to bereavement support groups. Professionals specifically trained and sensitive to bereavement and HIV-related issues may add a sense of safety to the group. By facilitating communication and preventing personal attack, professional facilitators may make it easier for clients to express the full of range of emotions. Bereavement support groups, even those that are professionally led, differ from psychotherapy groups in the assumption that members are basically psychologically healthy, and so diagnoses and individualized treatment plans are not used.

Sandra Jacoby Klein's book, *Heavenly Hurts: Surviving AIDS Related Deaths and Losses*, demonstrates the power of AIDS bereavement support groups led by competent mental health professionals.[93] While at times, leaders take an active facilitation role in their groups, at other times, as demonstrated in the following description, the mere presence of a watchful trained leader allows a level of disclosure that might otherwise be too intense for participants: this presence ensures participants that things will not get out of hand. By setting ground rules of acceptable behavior, the leader, in Klein's words, "creates an environment of safety and acceptance."

> *One mourner in a mixed group was a mother whose son had died of AIDS-related illness. She came to the group in deep grief and with great anger. The anger was frequently directed at the gay men in the group. For two sessions they just listened to her and didn't even discuss their grief. By the third session, Henry couldn't take it anymore. He exploded at her, yelling, "My grief is as great for my lover as yours is for your son. We all have a lot of grief and we are all angry too. So, its about time you listened to us!" The two of them went at each other yelling and crying. Everyone else was stunned by the outburst. As the session neared its end the two of them stared at each other in stony silence.*
>
> *We thought we'd never see either of them again but they both came to the next session. She started talking about how she never understood her son and wished he wasn't gay so he'd still be alive. Henry started talking about how his mother never understood him either. At times during the next several sessions they began dialoging with each other, hugging each other, and having coffee after the group meetings. They*

subsequently supported each other as adoptive mother and son for a long period. Having a safe environment to explore their relationship with their son and lover, as well as with each other, allowed them to come to a mutual understanding that was supportive to both of them. The other group members were also able to work out issues with their own parents by observing and sharing in the conversations. This particular mixed group was quite successful. We decided that the most important element to a successful group was the level of comfort we as therapists have with our decisions. We create an environment of safety and acceptance, and then participants will feel welcome.

While proficiency in managing intense emotional expression is one advantage of having a professional leader, knowing how to fold bereavement educational material into the group is also important. The combination of bereavement education and support can be accomplished through structured lectures or by highlighting educational points during the group discussion. A hypothetical interaction between Maria, a Latina woman grieving for three months the loss of her husband, and Sarah Thomas, a social worker, demonstrates the integration of bereavement education into a support group.

Maria: *Yesterday, I finally opened Ricardo's closet. I've dreaded doing that for these past three months. I was so afraid that I would be confronted with the smell of him on his clothes.*

Sarah: *What happened, how did you feel?*

Maria: *Yes, his smell was still there. A lot less than when I put his things away right after he died, but it was still there. I fell to the floor, a mess; it brought it all back to me so strongly, like it happened yesterday. I don't know when I will ever be able to remove his clothes, and I can't imagine ever being in love again.*

Sarah: *At times it feels like this pain will never go away. You miss him so much. Remember when we talked about the processes and tasks of grief? It seems to me that yesterday you began to experiment with the third task: adjusting your life to Ricardo not being there. This takes time. And I know there is a part of you that doesn't want to give up your beloved. It seems to me that you are trying to figure out in your own way how to keep Ricardo's memory alive, while moving on with your own life. Would anyone else like to say anything to Maria?*

Bereavement Risk Reduction Counseling

Bereavement risk reduction counseling – both individual and group – focuses on mitigating factors that place mourners at risk for bereavement distress. Mourners at risk may be identified through a variety of venues – ranging from the medical and mental health milieu to the home – through formal or informal risk assessment. This assessment needs to take into consideration both bereavement burdens and personal impediments to coping. (See Table 2: Risk Factors for AIDS Bereavement Distress in Chapter Two.)

While empirically validated bereavement prediction models do not exist and common sense and clinical judgment are still paramount, the risk factors delineated in Chapter Two serve as a guide for identifying mourners at risk. As mentioned previously, clinicians need to remember that single factors typically do not predict specific negative bereavement outcomes. Concern should be heightened by both the magnitude of each risk factor and the overall number of risk factors.

Once a clinician identifies a mourner as being at risk for bereavement distress, he or she should teach specific coping-oriented strategies to mitigate or eliminate the relevant risk factor. While risk reduction counseling is basically a preventive method, in combination with other forms of grief-related psychotherapy, it may aid mourners with complicated grief by reducing the risk for further complications.

A range of individual and small group counseling strategies can assist mourners in addressing specific risk factors. Research on the effectiveness of small groups in preventing bereavement complications has shown that interventions are most successful when they target mourners who demonstrate specific risk factors or high levels of distress. Other research stresses the importance of the timing of the intervention: intervening too soon, that is, within the first couple of weeks after loss, may have no positive effects or, as illustrated in one study, may even delay or interfere with the bereavement process.[82] Risk reduction strategies are problem-specific and time-limited. This type of counseling should be conducted by professional counselors or skilled volunteers trained specifically in bereavement risk reduction strategies.

Counseling to Reduce the Risk of Bereavement Distress

As discussed in Chapter Two, bereavement burdens are specific demands placed on the mourner, and personal impediments reflect characteristics or ongoing problems that interfere with the mourner's ability to cope with these burdens. Preventive interventions are designed to assist mourners in addressing these two types of risk factors prior to the onset of negative bereavement outcomes, and these interventions may be instituted even prior to an HIV-related death in the form of bereavement education and counseling.

The bereavement burdens listed in Chapter Two represent at least two types of burdens: status burdens and situational burdens. Status burdens, such as being HIV seropositive, having experienced multiple losses, or having been a caregiver, primary partner, parent, or spouse of a deceased person, cannot be changed by an intervention. However, status burdens may influence the type of interventions appropriate for a mourner. For example, specialized groups may be formed for seropositive mourners, parents, or spouses. Situational burdens, such as financial difficulties or interpersonal conflicts, may respond to more active interventions, for example, improving coping skills, such as problem-solving, decision making, or communication.

The bereavement burdens placed on a mourner as a result of his or her being seropositive may vary to a large degree depending upon the stage of HIV disease progression, the quality of social support, and financial resources. In some cases, social service planning prior to the death is required to augment financial and housing resources that may be reduced by the death of a roommate or life partner. Clinicians must avoid making assumptions related to needs of seropositive mourners. In response to the success of new medical regimens, many seropositive individuals are more optimistic about the future, and inferences about the inevitability of a seropositive mourner's decline may be clumsy. On the other hand, some seropositive individuals may find it difficult to initiate discussion of their own health concerns in the wake of a close friend's or partner's death. In general, it is wise to begin with a discussion of grief-related issues and then gently inquire as to an individual's view of his or her own health status. For example, a clinician may ask, "Has [the deceased's] death brought up thoughts and feelings about your own health status?"

Another common bereavement burden that may require risk reduction counseling is multiple loss or "bereavement overload."[8] Many mourners come to counseling feeling overwhelmed by the number of losses they have experienced and may need assistance organizing their bereavement to focus on the most important losses. Others may need to separate losses in order to fully grieve each.

Counselors should listen for hidden or unacknowledged losses, such as the sense of diminished freedoms or the loss of enjoyable sexual activities. Sometimes the fatigue of grief, in part due to the extended nature of the epidemic, wears individuals down and the suggestion of taking a "bereavement holiday" to focus on other matters for a period of time is welcomed by them.

Individuals come to the tasks of grieving with different levels of personal coping competency and personal problems. Research on predicting success in bereavement consistently suggests that an individual's pre-existing ability to cope with stress is the best predictor of bereavement outcome. The UCSF Coping Project found that in a sample of seropositive gay men who provided care to partners with HIV disease, those men who were able to maintain a fighting spirit, to cognitively reframe stress in terms of personal growth, to sustain adequate social support, and to plan a course of action were less depressed and had higher self-esteem.[27] Other research suggests the harmful effects of interpersonal conflict, ruminative thinking, excessive self-focus, and pessimism.[76] Counseling strategies to improve the outlook of mourners and their abilities to cope are crucial.

Recent Developments in AIDS Bereavement Coping Groups

Two models of group counseling to reduce the burdens and increase coping effectiveness for AIDS bereavement have recently been developed and evaluated. The first, called Coping Effectiveness Training, was designed by the UCSF Coping Project and is based on the cognitive theory of stress and coping.[94] The second approach, developed by the Center for AIDS Intervention Research (CAIR) of the Medical College of Wisconsin,[95] applies similar coping enhancement strategies, yet gives additional attention to group support and emotional expression. Both approaches have fared well in small pilot studies, improving coping, reducing depression, and increasing morale.

In Coping Effectiveness Training, group participants are taught a strategy for choosing among coping approaches to maximize effectiveness in managing bereavement burdens and reducing bereavement distress. In line with the Coping Project's definition of stress, project clinicians focus on two processes they feel mediate stress: appraisal and coping. In an approach developed by the project, clinicians teach participants to fit the coping strategy to the characteristics of the stressful situation. In other words, if a mourner has a solvable problem, such as financial difficulties or interpersonal conflict, clinicians encourage "problem-oriented coping" strategies. On the other hand, for clients responding emotionally to situations outside of their control, clinicians teach "emotion-focused coping," for example, relaxation techniques or positive distraction.[94]

The Coping Project protocol consists of a training phase and a maintenance phase. The training phase includes ten weekly two-hour sessions, with a day-long retreat between the fourth and fifth sessions. After the training phase, participants meet as a group every two months for the remainder of one year in order to maintain the training's effects. The training covers the following elements: appraisal of stressful situations; cognitive-behavioral approaches to problem-oriented and emotion-focused coping; appraisal-coping fit; the use of social support; and self-efficacy and maintenance training. The skills that comprise emotion-focused coping include cognitive restructuring, relaxation, and humor. The strategies that comprise problem-focused coping include problem-solving, social and communication skills, decision-making, and negotiation.

An interesting confluence exists between Coping Effectiveness Training and group strategies that use the 12-step model. Coping Effectiveness Training teaches participants to make appraisals based on the changeability of stressful situations. It encourages the use of problem-focused coping in situations in which the individual has a reasonable chance to effect change. On the other hand, it applies adaptive emotion-focused coping primarily with respect to unchangeable aspects of situations. This same idea is reflective in the 12-step program through the serenity prayer: "God grant me the serenity to accept the things I cannot change, the courage to change the things I can, and the wisdom to know the difference."[96]

Kathleen Sikkema and her colleagues at the Center for AIDS Intervention Research developed a variation of Coping Effectiveness Training that more explicitly combines supportive interventions with cognitive-behavioral approaches. For example, in the first session each participant presents his or her personal story or situation. These personal introductions include a description of the participant's relationship to the person(s) lost to AIDS, current difficulties and needs, and desired changes in coping with grief. Based on these disclosures, the facilitator highlights the uniqueness and universality of AIDS-related bereavement and identifies the group's goals and purposes.[95]

The facilitator further encourages participants to express their emotions related to loss and to learn ways to find expression for these emotions – such as talking with a friend or hitting a cooking pan – outside of the group setting. In the goal-setting phase of the group, with the help of the facilitator, members establish for themselves appropriate levels for their participation in community activities.

Psychotherapy for Complicated Grief

This section focuses on individual psychotherapeutic approaches to address issues of complicated grief. It describes two major variations of grief-related psychotherapy: problem-oriented approaches and psychodynamic approaches. Problem-oriented approaches emphasize specific behavioral changes to relieve the pain of complicated grief. A variety of behavioral and cognitive strategies – including the therapeutic use of grief rituals – are applied to this type of grief work. Psychodynamic approaches view complicated grief as blocked or unresolved grief and attempt to assist the client in understanding and resolving the underlying reasons for the blockage.

As discussed earlier, complicated grief is defined in this monograph by the following experience: a disruption in the course of grief characterized by an atypical intensity (overly numbed or overly intrusive) or duration (absent or chronic) of grief symptoms (shock, yearning, searching, disorganization, despair) that leads to an unacceptable duration of functional impairment in critical areas of work and relations. Further, while there is considerable overlap between the symptoms of complicated grief and psychiatric disorders – such as depression, post-traumatic stress disorder, and other anxiety disorders – clinicians are encouraged to make a differential diagnosis between these two types of conditions. This differential diagnosis allows clinicians to consider and prescribe appropriate psychotropic medications.

In selecting the appropriate type of bereavement psychotherapy, several factors need to be considered, including the level of psychological functioning of the mourner prior to bereavement and whether therapy is initiated early or later in the mourning process. Research conducted by Mary Vachon suggests that shortly after a death, mourners require therapeutic strategies that help them deal with inner distress and find meaning in the loss; later in the course of grief, mourners need to learn new roles and socialization. Research also suggests that supportive therapy is more likely to benefit clients with poorer functioning or lower motivation, while exploratory forms of therapy, including psychodynamic interpretations, are more likely to benefit highly motivated and psychologically minded clients.[97]

Problem-Oriented Grief Therapy

Time-limited, problem-oriented psychotherapy – focused on facilitating the tasks of grieving and on mitigating any risk factors – may be helpful to clients experiencing complicated grief, with or without co-existing mental disorders. Shuchter and Zisook suggest that rather than viewing the goal of bereavement therapy as the resolution of psychological attachment to the deceased, which may take several years, grief therapy should address specific grief-related problems with the understanding that the client can return if additional problems arise in the later stages of bereavement. Shuchter and Zisook developed a multidimensional approach to assessing and treating problems arising from spousal bereavement. This approach is problem-specific and addresses specific therapeutic tasks.[86]

One useful problem-oriented strategy is the therapeutic use of rituals. A grief ritual is a formal activity that provides a structure – a time and a place to honor an important loss. Therese Rando cites the benefits of using ritual to enhance grief psychotherapy with mourners who experience either psychic numbing or who are overwhelmed by grief.[98] Counselors can assist mourners to develop their own rituals or encourage the application of rituals prescribed by religious or cultural traditions. Bereavement rituals can also be included in group or individual counseling formats. When used in groups, rituals with universal themes are more appropriate. For example, many groups use rituals to elicit memories at the beginning of the session and to encourage redirection of focus away from grief at the end of the session.

Rituals may be particularly useful for clients blocked in their awareness and expression of grief since rituals may create a safe context in which to prompt memories and their associated emotions. For clients having difficulty modulating the strong intrusions of memories or images, rituals may help to limit these unwanted intrusions by providing a specific time and place for experiencing such painful mental phenomena. Through rituals, some depressed clients may combat the sense of helplessness that may accompany mourning, and angry clients may find a legitimate forum in which to express their feelings. Counselors can assist ruminative clients devise rituals that alter self-focus and encourage outward directed activities such as viewing art or observing nature. These strategies not only provide respite from anguish, but also teach clients that they can have control over the focus of their attention.

Rituals may be conducted once to emphasize a particular moment in time or they may be used on an ongoing basis. Regular rituals, such as a daily time for reflection, may enhance a mourner's understanding of the meaning and nature of loss, and this may help resolve his or her grief. Rituals with specific therapeutic targets may be used by counselors and therapists to assist clients reach therapeutic goals.

Psychodynamic Grief Therapy

Mardi Horowitz has developed and studied a time-limited (twelve sessions) psychodynamic grief psychotherapy model to assist people with complicated mourning.[32] According to this model, in the aftermath of any stressful life event, certain processes must occur to facilitate assimilation, accommodation, and healthy resumption of living. Individuals must resolve the personal meanings of the stressful event, including its implications for relationships, self-image, and behavior. This process entails the individual's reappraising the event and revising core models of self, role relationships, and future plans. Horowitz calls these core models of self and others "person schemata."

The primary goal of psychodynamic grief therapy is symptom reduction. This is accomplished through the mitigation of an individual's need for psychological defenses against awareness of ideas and images that lead to stress and intolerable emotional states. Therapy accomplishes this goal by helping mourners consciously connect their thoughts and memories of the stressful event with their associated emotional responses. For clients who tend to "overcontrol" their awareness of their inner life, and who thus experience emotional numbing, the therapeutic task is to encourage a re-experiencing of grief; for those who experience intrusive-repetitive thoughts or affects, the task is to promote avoidance or the working through of these painful phenomena. One technique Horowitz describes as a way to give clients a sense of mastery over emotions is called "dosing," a process that entails re-experiencing an event and its meanings for a specific time, putting it out of mind for a period, and again recalling the event.

According to Horowitz, complicated grief is the result of maladaptive habitual controls over ideas and feelings related to the self and others. The assumption is that complicated grief – in his terms, "blocked," "inhibited," or "chronic" – reflects the presence of unintegrated, unconscious or partially conscious, and contradictory views of the deceased or earlier relationships. One of the tasks of therapy, therefore, is to identify the emotions and evaluations associated with the deceased, and this will assist the mourner to come to terms with unresolved feelings. This type of exploratory work may also uncover other unresolved losses in the client's past that may need attention. Through this process of discovery, clients begin to better understand their schemata – their habitual views of themselves and others.

Horowitz developed a phase model of grief that is consistent with other stress response syndromes. His model includes the following phases: outcry, denial, intrusions, working-through, and completion. Each phase is assumed to reflect the activation of schemata and working models that organize the individual's dominant states of mind during mourning. Horowitz's model provides a method for analysis of the discrepancies between new schemata that may arise as the result of a recent loss and more enduring schemata. For example, the death of a husband may require a woman to revamp a major relationship schema: that of "wife." At first overwhelmed by all that this entails, she cries out in anguish. This stimulates her psychological defenses – psychologically pushing this conflict out of awareness – which leaves her feeling "gray" and "numb." As her defenses weaken, intrusive images or memories related to this loss of self-concept break through into her consciousness and bring to the surface painful emotions, such as fear, sadness, or anger. Provided she has the requisite ego strength to juggle the need to both tolerate these painful memories and to appropriately distract herself from them, she will be able to work through her grief and reorganize her relationship schemata. Her new view of herself is that of "widow," with all the meanings that go along with that identity.

The death of a loved one may also activate early schemata of the self as helpless, weak, childlike, inadequate, incapable, destructive, or evil. These "latent self-images" are assumed to form early in life as a consequence of some form of trauma.[99] As the individual matures, he or she learns more adaptive and compensatory concepts of self and other, and these dominate the personality. In addition, the supportive context of the relationship with the deceased may also have checked these latent negative self-images.[100] This aspect of Horowitz's model is particularly helpful in understanding the return of internalized homophobic thoughts and feelings by gay men who may have lived for years holding more positive views of themselves and other homosexuals. Working through these latent self images, may, in fact, have long ranging benefits to these gay men, who are further freed from the danger of their re-emergence in the future.

For all the phases of grief except completion – outcry, denial, intrusion, and working through – Horowitz identified normal and pathological responses, which typically comprised an intensification of the normal variant.[41] For example, during the outcry phase, the normal response is an outcry of emotion, while the pathological response may be panic. For the denial phase, the normal response is the avoidance of reminders and social withdrawal, while the pathological response may be substance abuse. For the intrusive phase, the normal response is recollecting negative experiences with the deceased, while the pathological response may be a flooding with negative images.

Therapists intervene at the points in these phases where mourning appears to be suspended. For example, if an individual is in a denial phase, the goal would be to facilitate greater emotional expression. If the individual is in an intrusive phase, the goal is to help the client modulate his or her emotions and to encourage an exploration of their meaning. Interventions of this type should free the individual to move toward fuller completion of the mourning.[100]

Psychiatric and Medical Intervention

In order to respond to bereavement distress, providers must determine the relationship between grief, mental disorder, and any physical disease. A thorough assessment, including a careful history of physical and psychiatric symptoms, is crucial to identifying preexisting disorders or vulnerabilities to disorder.

Although it is important to encourage mourners to experience grief, some people may become emotionally overwhelmed and may need assistance to tolerate intense grief. Whenever possible, clinicians should apply nonpharmacological interventions such as general relaxation exercises to reduce stress or behavioral approaches to reduce insomnia. When these approaches are not sufficient, judicious use of anti-anxiety agents and sleeping medications may be indicated. [101]

The use of psychotropic medications in the clinical management of bereavement is an area of great debate. Given the historic misuse of medication to "calm" mourners – especially women – there is general suspicion about this approach among bereavement experts.[37] According to Sidney Zisook, "Although some might argue that the use of psychotropic medications during bereavement is maladaptive in that these substances prevent the bereaved from 'getting in touch with their true feelings' and thereby block the resolution of grief, this position has not been validated by empirical data."[102]

Rando contends that failure to recognize and respect the reality that some mourners require psychotropic medication is as detrimental as forcing medication without just cause. She suggests that a treatment plan should include a careful medical examination as well as appropriate psychological and pharmacologic management. If clinicians suspect that medication is suppressing or interfering with grief, they should reconsider this approach, keeping in mind at all points that medication is an adjunct to psychological treatment and social support, not a replacement for them.[37]

According to Stephen Shuchter, it is important to conceptualize correctly the purposes of psychopharmacologic interventions with the bereaved.[103] He suggests, "Broadly speaking there are two kinds of circumstances for which these agents should be considered: treating co-morbid psychiatric conditions and modifying affects that are unique to the grief experience. With regard to the former, it becomes important to make diagnoses such as major depression, panic disorders, [and] obsessive-compulsive disorders . . . because if untreated, they will have untoward effects upon grief: they are likely to distort or exaggerate that process." In this context, grief needs to be treated as any other stress-precipitated disorder.

Shuchter further points out that pharmacological intervention for affective states that are transient to grief is much more controversial, has been little studied, and tends to reflect the philosophies of individual providers. In general, whenever behavioral mechanisms can be used to modify the level of anguish, they are desirable. The goal of desensitizing a client to images, affects, and other triggers of complicated grief reactions is critical. However, those clients who feel "tortured" by grief may require brief periods of medication. Furthermore, given the biological importance of sleep, it is appropriate to medicate sleep disturbances, even in the absence of other evidence of a "disorder."[103]

An Integrated Therapy for AIDS Bereavement

The final section of this monograph articulates the last element of the Integrative Model: an integrated approach to therapy for AIDS bereavement distress. The goal of this integrated approach to therapy reflects the aim of the whole Integrative Model, that is, to help AIDS mourners adequately manage the mourning process and to find a meaningful resolution to their grief. It does so by harnessing the techniques of psychotherapy and risk reduction counseling to assist mourners in successfully moving through the phases and tasks of mourning in a manner that is consistent with their personal and cultural values. For mourners whose grief is complicated, it seeks to modulate the intensity and duration of grief symptoms such as shock, yearning, disorganization, and despair; to reduce functional impairment in critical areas of work and relationship; and to reduce symptoms of clinical disorder such as depression, anxiety, guilt, and suicidal ideation.

To achieve these goals and guide therapy, the integrated approach applies four tasks: establishing rapport and validating loss; developing an integrative and dynamic understanding; working through psychodynamic blocks and facilitating cognitive and behavioral change; and reinforcing positive changes and terminating the therapy. While these tasks imply a general sequence of treatment and help clinicians set a reasonable clinical course, they cannot be applied rigidly. As therapy progresses, it may require a temporary or permanent refocus on different tasks.

Task I. Establishing Rapport and Validating the Loss

As is true for most effective therapeutic approaches, the first task of Integrative AIDS Bereavement Therapy is to listen carefully to the client's story. By responding in an empathic manner that acknowledges and validates the client's experience, the clinician establishes rapport. A sympathetic review of details of the client's relationships and the events that led up to and followed the death also helps the client understand the meaning of the death for him or her. Through this exploration and a careful discussion of the goals and expectations of the therapy, the clinician and the client forge a collaborative working relationship.

Task II. Developing an Integrative and Dynamic Understanding

The second task of Integrative AIDS Bereavement Therapy is to determine the type and level of bereavement distress and the psychological factors affecting the mourning process.

Assess for Complicated Grief. The clinician and the client review the client's progress through the course (phases and tasks) of grief, the intensity and duration of grief symptoms, the nature of grief symptoms, and the level of functional disruption. Taking into account the client's individual and cultural values, the clinician and client then determine whether the client is suffering complicated grief. If so, clinician and client explore the possibility of conscious or unconscious conflicts and mechanisms that may be blocking the mourning process.

Assess for Clinical Disorder. Using standard diagnostic procedures,[36] the clinician and client review mental and physical symptoms and previous psychiatric history to uncover co-existing clinical disorders and to evaluate the need for psychopharmacological intervention.

Assess Bereavement Risk Factors. The clinician assesses bereavement burden and personal impediments to coping to determine whether specific cognitive or behavioral changes are required to improve coping. If so, the client and clinician collaborate to prioritize goals and develop programs to reduce bereavement burden and increase coping skills.

Task III. Working Through Psychodynamic Blocks and Facilitating Behavioral Change

Based on the assessment in Task II, the clinician and client establish specific therapeutic goals and strategies to meet those goals. These strategies may include: using bereavement education to support the client, to increase his or her knowledge, and to reduce his or her alienation; analyzing further and working through psychodynamic blocks to grief resolution; and setting cognitive or behavioral goals and programs to reduce bereavement burden and increase coping skills.

As demonstrated earlier in this chapter, bereavement education can assist clients both to structure their expectations and goals, and to reinforce their progress toward resolving grief. Other therapeutic activities to support this task of working through blocks and facilitating change may include helping clients to restructure their self-concepts and self-esteem, identify and express emotions, communicate more effectively, address specific problems, and make new life decisions. The clinician serves as a guide for structuring the sessions, and as an empathic and inquiring listener, a confronter of inconsistencies, an encourager and motivator, an interpreter of underlying psychodynamics, and an expert in behavioral change. He or she may use activities such as therapeutic rituals to provide a structure for change. Working together, the client and clinician determine how to allocate their time – both during the session and over the course of the therapy.

Adjunct community resources may enhance and augment therapy. These resources may include community-wide AIDS ceremonies and rituals, AIDS bereavement support groups, AIDS bereavement risk reduction classes, and a variety of resources that assist clients improve social support, meet new people, and find meaning in their lives.

Task IV. Reinforcing Positive Changes and Terminating Therapy

At the end of therapy, a brief termination period provides time for the client and clinician to review lessons learned and to reinforce any cognitive and behavioral changes. This period also allows client and clinician time to debrief the therapeutic process in order to consider how specific changes may relate to other aspects of the client's life, and to process therapeutic termination, which may rekindle feelings of loss.

Successful mourning is dependent on a range of individual factors, and its achievement may require the mourner to return to therapy for further assistance and reinforcement after the termination of initial therapy. Given the continuity of goals and dynamics within these therapeutic episodes, each episode may be considered a phase in an ongoing therapeutic process, and phases may be separated by varying periods of time. Bereaved clients may return to therapy some time after termination, for example, as they move into a new phase of grief or on the occasion of an anniversary, which may bring back a confusing intensification of grief. The return may last only a few sessions, reinforcing previously achieved progress, or it may extend, depending on the complexity of the issues raised.

On the other hand, integrated AIDS bereavement therapy may require a significant change in focus after the initial grief work has been finished. As seen in the following case example, after uncovering longer-standing personality issues, therapy may require a change in direction, the restatement of goals, and the application of different therapeutic strategies.

Integrative Therapy: The Case of Paul

The case of Paul offers insights into how to apply Integrative AIDS Bereavement Therapy. It follows a client through the course of initial therapy and re-evaluation, into a second phase of therapy, and finally to the termination of therapy. Paul, a forty-year-old gay man, was referred for bereavement therapy by his physician, who was treating him for migraine headaches. He started therapy with Henry

Garrison, PhD three months after the death of David, his partner of nine years. Paul was the son of a wealthy family who owned a large lumber company with branches throughout the state.

Paul described a highly conflicted relationship with his family and the family business, which was now run by his older brother. He had served many functions in the business, including a disastrous stint as a store manager shortly after he graduated high school, which required him to return to the home office for additional training. He then took over the store that he had managed when he met David. After the death of his father, Paul left the business altogether to become a "house husband," but returned when David went on disability: "We began to get on each others nerves – always being together." At the time he entered therapy, Paul was working in a low-level position in the warehouse, as he put it, "It keeps me busy, but doesn't tax me too much."

In the first session, Paul recounted the story of David's death. "After three years with AIDS, David had taken a turn for the worse. The doctor diagnosed *Mycobacterium avium* complex, treated it, and assured us that David would recover. On the day before David's death, I had had a rough time tending to him and I decided to sleep on the couch. David protested a bit, but I insisted that I needed the rest. The next day, I found David on the floor next to our bed – his body contorted and dead." Since that morning, this image of David had haunted Paul.

Paul had served as David's primary caregiver throughout his illness. Over the three or four months before his death, David's need for care had become intense, requiring Paul to orchestrate many visits to doctors' offices, take on most of the household chores, and attend to David's emotional and nursing needs. Paul was an enthusiastic caregiver and jealously protected his time with David – at times refusing help from family and friends. David returned from a short stay in the hospital several days before his death, a return that was both joyful and burdensome for Paul. It was the fatigue from this homecoming that motivated Paul to sleep alone on the night of David's death.

During the first few days after David's death, Paul carried out the many activities of notifying friends and family, and making arrangements for David's cremation. Paul's mood vacillated between a strange calm and gnawing anxiety. As he put it, "Things didn't seem real; I felt like I was walking in a dream." Along with the shock of finding David's body, Paul felt exhaustion from the overwhelming demands of David's illness and death. Paul had difficulty falling asleep and staying asleep and took sleeping medication prescribed by his physician every night during his first three weeks of mourning. When he was able to sleep, he dreamed the recurring nightmare of finding David's body.

Weeks after the death, Paul began to register its reality and to feel both pangs of intense pining and a great restlessness. When he experienced the image of the death scene, Paul tried desperately to push it away and the guilt and remorse he associated with it. At times, he felt David's presence in the room and was startled to hear himself call out to David. Paul's nights were filled with vivid dreams of David – alive and dead – and Paul often woke in a panic, fearing that he had forgotten to do something for David. Paul described becoming enraged by small inconveniences, such as waiting in line or driving, experiences that were followed by deep sobbing. He noticed himself searching through the crowds, not exactly sure what he was looking for, until he realized he was longing to see David just one more time.

As a co-owner in the family business, Paul was able to take off as much time as he needed to deal with his grief. When he returned to work after three weeks, he arranged his schedule to allow himself to work odd hours, usually alone. While he had the energy to work each day, he had little left for anything else, and he felt estranged from family and friends. Paul was often annoyed with his family – feeling sometimes that their concern for him was intrusive and at other times that they were not distressed enough over David's death. At first Paul tried to visit old haunts, but usually he left abruptly when his sense of loss became too intense. Finally, he began to avoid places that reminded him of David, spending most of his free time "staring at the boob tube."

Three months after David's death, at the time of his first session with Dr. Garrison, Paul suffered frequently from moderate to severe anxiety and pervasively from mild to moderate depression. He was still using sleep medication three or four nights a week and had nightmares almost every night. He had difficulty falling asleep and would wake early in the morning unable to return to sleep. He had migraine headaches two to three times per week. He spent a large amount of time ruminating about the last scene of David's life, asking himself repeatedly why had he slept on the couch that night. Although Paul understood that he been a devoted – even doting – lover, the guilt associated with this final event threatened to negate all the love that went before. Paul also remained isolated from friends and family.

Initial Assessment

Applying Tasks I and II, during the first three sessions of therapy, Dr. Garrison established rapport through an empathic review of Paul's story and conducted an inquiry into Paul's grief and clinical symptoms. Using this information, Dr. Garrison determined whether Paul was suffering from complicated grief or clinical disorders and whether he was experiencing any risks for bereavement distress.

Uncomplicated versus Complicated Grief

While Paul was perplexed to some degree by the intensity of symptoms and was bothered by intrusive images, he understood his need to grieve. He also understood how central David had been in his life, and the intensity of his grief appeared to be consistent with the level of this loss. As a practicing Catholic, Paul believed that a mourning period of one year was typical and he was not concerned about the duration of his grief symptoms. Dr. Garrison acknowledged the value of this insight in terms of recognizing the normality of Paul's grief within the context of his personal and cultural background. Dr. Garrison was, however, concerned about the intensity of Paul's symptoms and the degree to which the longing, searching, disorganization, and despair interfered with Paul's ability to get social support. Of greater concern was the vividness and frequency of intrusive images of the death scene and Paul's accompanying guilt and diminished self-esteem. Dr. Garrison gave Paul a provisional diagnosis of complicated mourning.

Grief versus Clinical Disorder

In the early stages of mourning, it is difficult to differentiate grief – complicated or uncomplicated – from depression, PTSD, and other anxiety disorders. Using diagnostic procedures outlined in the DSM-IV, Dr. Garrison noted that, consistent with major depression, Paul experienced depressed mood, markedly diminished interest in and pleasure from activities, insomnia, exhaustion, diminished ability to concentrate, and marked social withdrawal. Paul qualified for all four PTSD criteria:

- *Exposure:* He was exposed to a traumatic event that involved an actual death, and he responded with fear, helplessness, and horror.
- *Re-Experiencing Trauma*: He persistently re-experienced the trauma through recurrent and intrusive distressing recollections of the death scene, had distressful dreams, and reacted emotionally and physiologically to cues that reminded him of finding David's body.

- *Avoidance*: Frequently, he could not sleep in the bedroom in which he found David and he withdrew emotionally into a state of psychic numbness.
- *Increased Arousal:* He exhibited symptoms of increased arousal – difficult sleep, irritability, and frequent outbursts of anger.

Finally, consistent with other anxiety disorders, Paul demonstrated excessive physical anxiety symptoms – shaking, sweaty hands, and muscle tension – mental tension, and frequent ruminative thinking.

Given the magnitude of the symptoms – which were mitigated by how recent the death was – Dr. Garrison made a provisional diagnosis of PTSD. He planned to re-evaluate this diagnosis three months later and deferred a secondary diagnosis of major depression, other anxiety disorder, or any personality disorder. Dr. Garrison made a provisional diagnosis of complicated bereavement. He further observed that Paul was suffering from migraine headaches, and noted bereavement and conflict with his family as major stressors.

AIDS Bereavement Risk Factor Assessment

Dr. Garrison identified several risk factors that could further exacerbate Paul's bereavement distress. Paul's bereavement burden was high: he had been the primary caregiver and had experienced tremendous demands that caused exhaustion. Paul also perceived inadequate social and emotional support, and experienced considerable conflict with his family. Further, Paul exhibited several personal impediments to coping: relatively poor coping skills and poor self-esteem.

Diagnosis and Treatment Plan

Dr. Garrison gave Paul a diagnosis of complicated mourning with a clinical disorder and considered him to be at high risk for prolonged bereavement distress. Paul agreed to an initial twelve sessions of Integrative AIDS Bereavement Therapy and to re-evaluation at the end. Therapy would focus on helping Paul understand the nature of his grief, manage grief symptoms, reduce bereavement burden, increase coping skills, and reduce anxiety, depression, and PTSD symptoms.

Initial Phase of Therapy

Task I. Establishing Rapport and Validating the Loss

During the early stages of therapy, Paul vacillated between emotional and social withdrawal and an outcrying of pain, intrusive memories, and guilt related to the way David died. He enjoyed recounting the story of the couple's relationship: how he had lavished attention on David, and how David, unlike previous lovers, had returned his love. He sobbed as he remembered how together they had worked their way out of alcohol and drug abuse, supporting each other in their recovery and their coming to terms with being gay. Paul reported the incidences related to David's seroconversion and illnesses with sadness and anguish mixed with a sense of pride in his own competence as a caregiver. Paul also felt proud that he had returned to the family business "on my terms," being helpful in small ways while not placing too great a demand on himself.

Since David's death, Paul often had imaginary conversations with him, when he wanted advice about how to manage social interactions or when he had difficulty controlling his emotions. He often remembered one of David's favorite lines when confronted by an aggressive driver, "You don't need to out-asshole the asshole." Remembering this soothed Paul and often allowed him to chuckle to himself and let go of his anger. During this time Dr. Garrison listened carefully and validated the enormity of Paul's loss. Through empathic responses to the full range of Paul's concerns, including descriptions of explicit sexual activities, Dr. Garrison gained Paul's trust and Paul began to discuss more freely his innermost thoughts and feelings, including his conflicted feelings regarding being gay.

Task II. Developing an Integrative and Dynamic Understanding

Dr. Garrison helped Paul understand what David's death meant to him. Not only was David his beloved partner, he also represented Paul's greatest successes: ending his career of substance abuse, learning that he could be a good lover, learning that it was possible to live honorably as a gay man. Furthermore, Paul began to see how much the partners relied on each other for advice and for help in managing their emotions. Now Paul needed to learn to do much of that for himself.

Paul described feeling stuck. On one hand, he knew that he needed to get on with his life; on the other hand, he fought any efforts to move him past his grief. Dr. Garrison educated Paul about the course and tasks of mourning, how mourning takes time, how the time it takes is different for each individual, how feelings of longing, yearning, and searching are normal. By helping Paul understand that the first tasks of grief were to accept the reality of the loss and experience the emotions of grief, Dr. Garrison gave Paul permission to express his deep sorrow and anger.

As the therapy entered its third month, Dr. Garrison began to help Paul see that his reactions to David's death were determined both by the immediate loss of David, and to some degree, by more long-standing beliefs and feelings about himself and others. Paul responded that he knew that he had long suffered from diminished self-esteem. In fact, he had always wanted help with this matter but feared that he was not up to the challenge of "facing his demons."

Task III. Working Through Psychodynamic Blocks and Facilitating Cognitive and Behavioral Change

In order to structure this early phase of intense grieving, Dr. Garrison and Paul discussed ways that Paul could "dose" his grief by spending a set amount of time each day with David's memory and then forcing himself to turn his attention elsewhere. Paul developed a ritual of spending ten to thirty minutes each morning – usually in the shower – talking with David, describing what he wanted to get accomplished that day, what he was going to do to honor David, what he was going to do for other people, and what he was going to do for himself. Dr. Garrison encouraged Paul to identify, experience, and validate the emotions that arose during these conversations. Dr. Garrison then taught Paul techniques to redirect his attention to other matters. He taught Paul to use cognitive "thought-stopping" techniques to identify and intentionally impede unconstructive ruminative thoughts and images of the death. Awareness exercises helped him reduce self-focus and to learn to externalize his attention away from disturbing mental phenomena. Finally, pleasurable activities acted as positive distracters. After several weeks, David followed through with Dr. Garrison's recommendation that he join a short-term AIDS bereavement group. He hoped this approach would reduce his isolation, give him the chance to witness others grappling with grief, and offer him support and validation.

Over the period of one month, Paul reported feeling more in control of his life and his emotions. His contacts with his family – his mother, older brother and sister, and younger brother – were more pleasant. With the encouragement of Dr. Garrison, Paul began to discuss with his family the kind of support that he wanted: that he did not want David to be forgotten. Paul reported a touching moment in which his mother asked to see some old family pictures of David with Paul's nieces and nephews. He cried with sorrow and joy when his nine-year-old niece told him how much she missed David and drew a picture of him. At the same time, Paul began to put limits on the amount of time he was willing to spend with his family. As he put it, "When David was alive I always had an out. I could just say that we had plans. That doesn't work so well without him."

Toward the middle of this phase of therapy, Paul began to discuss his early childhood. He described his family: an alcoholic father, who lived in the shadow of Paul's domineering grandfather and who left the family when Paul was in high school; a mother whose main concern was keeping up appearances; and two brothers and a sister known for their voracious competitiveness. He both took pride and felt deep sadness in recalling that all of the boys in the family – Dad included – were seen as eccentric, hard-drinking, and mischievous. He described his struggles during adolescence to cope with his emerging homosexuality, and his earlier beliefs that homosexuality was wrong and that all homosexuals are weak and untrustworthy. While Paul no longer believed these ideas, they returned to haunt him when he was at his weakest. Dr. Garrison reassured Paul by saying, "By bringing these previously suppressed thoughts and feelings to consciousness, you can begin to reduce their power over you."

During this time Paul's anxiety diminished considerably, however, he continued to have difficulty sleeping. Dr. Garrison educated Paul about the need for a regular sleep-wake cycle, and the two developed a sleep schedule. Paul initiated an exercise program and began listening to relaxation tapes in the evening. These activities had a moderately positive, but intermittent, effect on his sleep and anxiety.

Three-Month Re-Evaluation of Therapy

After three months Dr. Garrison and Paul evaluated the progress of therapy in terms of symptoms of complicated grief, clinical disorders, risk factor analysis, and the overall treatment plan.

Uncomplicated versus Complicated Grief

Paul felt he was moving through the phases and tasks of mourning adequately. While he continued to long for David – at times desperately – he felt less confused by these longings. He better understood the nature of his grief and believed that his mourning was proceeding on track. On the other hand, the intrusive images of the death scene continued to haunt him almost daily. While the structuring activities – dosing, cognitive thought-stopping, and awareness exercises – gave Paul some measure of control over these intrusive images, the images were still a source of anxiety and guilt. Dr. Garrison determined that even in light of Paul's progress, Paul continued to qualify for a diagnosis of complicated grief.

Grief versus Clinical Disorder

Paul continued to experience moderate anxiety and mild to moderate depression, characterized by depressed mood, lack of interest in activities, and frequent ruminative thinking. His sleep continued to be problematic, with sleep disruption requiring medication several nights per week. These symptoms, along with the intrusive images of the death scene, continued periods of social and emotional withdrawal, and regular periods of increased emotional and physical arousal led Dr. Garrison to confirm his diagnosis of PTSD, with a secondary diagnosis of major depression.

After three months observation, Dr. Garrison identified a pattern of personality deficits, which predated bereavement and was consistent with a diagnosis of personality disorder. Paul's long-standing negative self-concepts and self-esteem appeared to be exacerbated by his grief. He exhibited a tendency toward social inhibition, feelings of inadequacy, and hypersensitivity to negative evaluation, largely stemming from his childhood. He avoided additional work responsibilities and social opportunities for fear of being criticized. While his tendency to hypersensitivity to criticism was consistent with Avoidant Personality Disorder, the magnitude of this aspect of the problem did not appear to warrant that diagnosis. Dr. Garrison diagnosed Paul with a "personality disorder, not otherwise specified."

AIDS Bereavement Risk Factor Assessment

Over the course of several months, the exhaustion Paul had experienced as a caregiver abated. He was happier with his level of social support from his family, however, he remained fairly isolated from peers once his bereavement group had ended. He was especially lonely for contact with other gay men. While his sobriety seemed solid, Dr. Garrison had some concern that Paul might slip back into these negative coping mechanisms without ongoing therapeutic support. Paul appeared to have significant personal deficits in coping skills. Without his deceased partner's promptings and support, Paul had difficulty managing stressful situations.

Treatment Plan

Paul agreed to another eight months of therapy. The focus of the therapy would be three-fold: to better understand the causes and psychological mechanisms associated with Paul's poor self-esteem; to continue to reduce bereavement burden and increase coping skills; and to reduce symptoms of clinical anxiety, depression, and PTSD. Dr. Garrison suggested the eight-month period in order to assist Paul through the one-year anniversary of David's death, which would occur six months after this three-month evaluation. Furthermore, Dr. Garrison referred Paul for a psychiatric evaluation, and Paul eventually began taking the antidepressant medication, paroxetine (Paxil).

Second Phase of Therapy

The second phase of Paul's therapy expanded to include a deeper understanding of factors that affected his self-esteem and blocked the resolution of his grief. Dr. Garrison's efforts to attend to Paul and to respond with empathy yielded a deeper rapport and a willingness on Paul's part to delve further into his insecurities.

Task II. Developing an Integrative and Dynamic Understanding

During the second phase of therapy, Dr. Garrison and Paul spent more time discussing Paul's early life and the history of his relationship with David. Through appropriate questioning, Dr. Garrison encouraged Paul to review historical material relevant to his ongoing perceptions and evaluations of himself, others, and his relationships. Through compassionate confrontation and interpretation, Dr. Garrison helped Paul begin to see patterns of thinking, emotional responses, and behavior that limited his personal effectiveness.

As the weeks unfolded, Paul described more of his early life. His elementary school years were filled with fear and shame. "I was a little queer kid, terrible at sports, not good in school, and the brunt of a lot of jokes by the other kids. I decided that I would rather be known as a trouble-maker than a sissy, so I started getting into a lot of trouble." In fact, this pattern of mischief had a long tradition in Paul's family, dating to his father's rebellion against Paul's grandfather, who was the patriarch and founder of the family business. Paul spoke with a mixture of pride and embarrassment as he recounted boyhood pranks with his older brother such as sneaking off in the family car or burning down the neighbor's garage.

While Paul's mother became enraged by the boys' antics, his father would "rave a bit and then wink." On several occasions his father had to "buy off" the Catholic school he attended so it would take him back after flunking a class. Paul learned to see himself both as a "wise guy" and a "chip off the old block." More importantly, he had been left with grave doubts about his intellectual abilities and his ability to take care of himself. Beyond this, he had lived with intense shame and fear that someone would discover his sexual desires for other boys.

By the time Paul reached high school, he had a full-blown cocaine and alcohol problem. He was known as the "life of the party." While in retrospect, he understood that most of his friends either suspected or knew that he was gay, he felt that he needed to curry favor with the "cool crowd" by spending large sums of money, providing the other kids with drugs, and chauffeuring them around in his new car. In his junior year in high school, Paul became extremely depressed, partially due to his drug use and partially due to some early disappointing sexual explorations with other boys. One evening he decided to drive his car off the road. He remembered thinking, "If it killed me, so be it; if I lived, surely they would send me to get help." Fortunately, Paul was not badly hurt. Unfortunately, his parents, in the midst of a divorce, spent their efforts trying to keep the matter quiet, never sending him for the help he desperately needed and wanted, but was afraid to request.

After high school, Paul attended community college for one semester. When his grades were lackluster, his father told him that he didn't want to waste any more money on Paul's education and insisted that Paul join the family firm. Paul was both humiliated and relieved not to have to deal with school. The change also gave him plenty of "partying money." The next four or five years Paul calls the "lost years." Continuing to fulfill his family obligations – Christmas at his mother's house, golf with his dad, Easter with the family in Hawaii – he lived a highly "closeted life." Attracting many men who enjoyed his money and his cocaine, his belief that "gay men can not be trusted" was reinforced. All the while, he secretly harbored the hope that one day he would find a gay man who would love him for himself and would enjoy a simple domestic life. He realized that he really detested his self-destructive lifestyle: "I always wanted to do something good with my life."

When he was 29 years old and managing one of the family businesses, Paul hired David to be a salesman. Given that he was not officially "out" to his family or at work, Paul was reluctant to approach

David, even though he knew that David was gay. One evening, after working together late, he invited David out to dinner. That led to a hot weekend of sex and drugs. For the next few months, he tried not to respond to David's advances, but finally, Paul gave in to his desires, and the two began to spend most evenings together, usually having sex and doing drugs. Slowly, however, they began to do things other than get drunk and high. On the evening that Paul learned of the death of his father, David held and comforted him – neither was drunk nor stoned.

Over the next five years, Paul and David ended their drug and alcohol use completely. Shortly after his father's death, Paul decided to leave the family business for a period of time feeling that he no longer needed to comply with his father's wishes. He never liked the responsibility of being a boss, and secretly dreaded being criticized or being discovered as incompetent. During that time, David continued to work for the business, and Paul became a "house husband." This was the happiest time in his life. David helped Paul maintain good relations with the family while giving him an excuse not to be at their beck and call. Paul at last felt like a success: "Being a loving husband – I finally found something that I could do well." A couple of years later, when David went out on disability, Paul felt able to return to work in the warehouse on his own terms.

Task III. Working Through Psychodynamic Blocks and Facilitating Change

In undertaking the work of Task III during the second phase, Dr. Garrison and Paul continued the cognitive and behavioral program initiated in the first phase of therapy. Dr. Garrison helped Paul to use techniques for reducing intrusive cognitions, seek support and set limits with his family, maintain a proper sleep schedule, learn to relax through the use of relaxation tapes, and establish and maintain an exercise program. Additionally, Paul and Dr. Garrison worked to identify projects that would give Paul's life purpose. Having returned to work after David's disability, Paul became more involved with larger decisions related to the family business and began to participate in board meetings. He discussed wanting to return to school to finish his college degree, the lack of which was a source of great shame for him. As Paul set reasonable goals for himself, every week he and Dr. Garrison would review the ways in which he succeeded – or did not succeed – to meet them. Through this review, Paul learned to identify cognitive and emotional blocks to completing tasks, and, thus, to finding success.

As Paul recounted his relationship with David, a picture emerged of a man who had "lost his other half." Dr. Garrison helped Paul identify those psychological functions that David provided Paul and assisted him in devising ways to take responsibility for these functions himself. A dramatic example occurred about eight months into the therapy. On his way home from work one evening, a man driving a small pickup truck almost hit Paul's car. Enraged, Paul made an obscene gesture. The man rammed his car into Paul's and sped away. Paul followed in at high speed and then pulled off the freeway and called the highway patrol. Both Paul and the other driver were arrested for reckless driving. In discussing the incident, Paul lamented that had David been with him, Paul would not have lost his cool. He said, "This is an example of something I need to learn: how to calm myself down." In subsequent sessions, Paul spent a great deal of time developing an inner dialogue between his nurturing, self-disciplining aspect and his sad, scared, angry aspect.

Throughout the first year of Paul's mourning, his grief vacillated greatly. When other aspects of his life were going well, his grief seemed manageable; when he faced disappointments, he would re-experience a great longing for David. This longing became especially salient the month of the anniversary of David's death. Dr. Garrison and Paul spent a great deal of time in therapy discussing ways that Paul could "take care of himself" during this period. Paul arranged with his mother to spend time with him on the day after the anniversary. As he put it, "I want that day to be alone with David; the next day I'll spend with the family." On the anniversary day, he woke early and went to mass, lighting a candle for David. He took a walk on a deserted beach, allowing himself to cry and "rage at the sea." The following day he felt calmer than he had for a long time and more hopeful about the future.

Task IV. Reinforcing Positive Changes and Terminating Therapy

During the final months of therapy, the vacillation in Paul's grief continued, however, the intensity of the longing diminished considerably. Consistent with Worden's third task of grief, "Adjusting to an Environment in Which the Deceased is Missing," Paul began sorting through David's clothing and made plans to donate most of them to charity. He said, "I just couldn't give everything away, but I don't need a monument to David in my closet either." He noticed that it was easier for him to talk about David without the deep pangs of grief. He notified the management of his building that he would be interested in trading his current condominium for another one when it became available. Over the course of the last six months, he had begun going out more with gay friends and had even gone on a few dates.

Paul's depression and PTSD symptoms had been reduced considerably and were now mild. Although his sleep continued to be disturbed occasionally, it was greatly improved, allowing him to feel refreshed most days. The intrusive images of David's death scene were less frequent, less vivid and disturbing, and more amenable to refocusing. Paul's migraine headaches also appeared to have significantly diminished. Paul remained on his antidepressant medication and agreed to return for a medication review twice a year.

Dr. Garrison and Paul spent the last couple of months in therapy reinforcing positive cognitive and behavioral changes and reviewing situations that required Paul to soothe himself and control his emotional reactions. He felt proud of his accomplishments in "taking care of himself" and frequently chuckled as he reflected on what David might think of the advances that he had made. Paul ended therapy fourteen months after David's death. He knew that he could return to see Dr. Garrison if his depression or PTSD increased or if he needed help coping with life's burdens or the mourning process.

Conclusion: Resolving AIDS Grief

Whether on the community, small group, or individual level, the Integrative Model of AIDS Bereavement helps AIDS mourners seek support from friends and family, other mourners, and professional helpers. By differentiating four types and levels of bereavement distress, it leads to specific and effective strategies to assist these mourners. While formal assessment and treatment of AIDS bereavement distress requires a trained professional, the model offers guidance to anyone who seeks to assist AIDS mourners to find the help that they need.

The overall goal of the Integrative Model is to help AIDS mourners adequately manage the mourning process and find meaningful resolution to their grief. The intention of the model is to be broad enough to manage the universal aspects of bereavement, yet specific enough to address the uniqueness of individual AIDS mourners. Placed within a social, cultural, and historical context, the Integrative Model guides efforts to provide knowledgeable and compassionate care to all those who suffer the loss of a loved one to AIDS. In so doing, it benefits the healing process for both individuals and communities.

References

1. Stroebe MS, Stroebe W, Hansson RO. Bereavement research and theory: An introduction to the handbook. In Stroebe MS, Stroebe W, Hansson RO, eds. *Handbook of Bereavement: Theory, Research, and Intervention*. Cambridge: Cambridge University Press, 1993.
2. Anonymous personal communication, San Francisco, 1985.
3. Bateson MC, Goldsby R. *Thinking AIDS: The Social Response to the Biological Threat*. Reading, Mass.: Addison-Wesley Publishing Co., 1988.
4. Rofes E. *Reviving the Tribe: Sexuality and Culture in the Ongoing Epidemic*. New York: Harrington Park Press, 1996.
5. Kelly JA. *Changing HIV Risk Behavior: Practical Strategies*. New York: Guilford Press, 1996.
6. Summers J. Bereavement. In Smith R, ed. *Encyclopedia of AIDS*. Chicago: Fitzroy Dearborn Publishers, 1998.
7. Centers for Disease Control and Prevention. Update in trends in AIDS incidence, deaths, and prevalence – U.S. 1996. *Morbidity and Mortality Weekly Reports*. 1997; 46(8): 165-173.
8. Lennon MJ, Martin JL, Dean L. The influence of social support of AIDS-related grief reaction among gay men. *Social Science and Medicine*. 1990; 31(4): 477-484.
9. Kelly B, Raphael B, Ross M, et al. A comparison of the psychosocial aspects of AIDS and cancer-related bereavement. *International Journal of Psychiatry in Medicine*. 1996; 26(1): 35-49.
10. Parkes CM, Weiss RS. *Recovery from Bereavement*. New York: Basic Books, 1983.
11. Fullilove MT. Beyond stereotypes: Stigma and the counseling process. In Dilley JW, Marks R, eds. *The UCSF AIDS Health Project Guide to Counseling*. San Francisco: Jossey-Bass Publishers, 1998.
12. Charmatz K. *The Social Reality of Death*. Reading, Mass.: Addison-Wesley Publishing Co., 1980.
13. Metcalf P, Huntington R. *Celebrations of Death: The Anthropology of Mortuary Ritual*. Second Edition. Cambridge: Cambridge University Press, 1991.
14. Seeley J, Kajura EB. Grief and the community. In Sherr L, ed. *Grief and AIDS*. Chichester, U.K.: John Wiley and Sons, 1995.
15. Gant LM. HIV/AIDS caregivers in African-American communities: Contemporary issues. In Lynch VJ, Wilson PA. *Caring for the HIV/AIDS Caregiver*. Westport, Conn.: Auburn House, 1996.
16. Shernoff M. Introduction. In Shernoff M, ed. *Gay Widowers: Life After the Death of a Partner*. New York: Harrington Park Press, 1997.
17. Shernoff M. Gay widowers: Grieving in relation to trauma and social support. *Journal of the Gay and Lesbian Medical Association*. 1998; 2(1): 27-33.
18. Wortman CB, Silver RC, Kessler RC. The meaning of loss and adjustment to bereavement. In Stroebe MS, Stroebe W, Hansson RO, eds. *Handbook of Bereavement: Theory, Research, and Intervention*. Cambridge: Cambridge University Press, 1993.
19. Yalom ID. *Existential Psychotherapy*. New York: Basic Books, 1980.
20. Costello CL. Religion and AIDS-related bereavement: A study of partners and family members. *Dissertation Abstracts International*. 1993; 54(6B): 3335.

21. Price-Spratlen T. Tracing time. In Shernoff M, ed. *Gay Widowers: Life After the Death of a Partner*. New York: Harrington Park Press, 1997.
22. Mead C. Crisis of the Psyche: Psychotherapeutic considerations on AIDS, loss and hope. In Sherr L, ed. *Grief and AIDS*. Chichester, U.K.: John Wiley and Sons, 1995.
23. Sansevero L. Sharing the journey. *On Display: Newsletter of the NAMES Project Foundation*. 1998; 11(2): 5.
24. Freud S. Mourning and melancholia. In Strachey J, ed. and trans. *The Standard Edition of the Complete Psychological Works of Sigmund Freud*. Vol. 14. London: Hogarth Press, 1914.
25. Prigerson HG, Frank E, Kasl SV, et al. Complicated grief and bereavement-related depression as distinct disorders: Preliminary empirical validation in elderly bereaved spouses. *American Journal of Psychiatry*. 1995; 152(1): 22-30.
26. Zisook S, DeVaul RA, Click MA. Measuring symptoms of grief and bereavement. *American Journal of Psychiatry*. 1982; 139(12): 1590-1593.
27. Folkman S, Chesney M, Collette L, et al. Postbereavement depressive mood and its prebereavement predictors in HIV-positive and HIV-negative men. *Journal of Personality and Social Psychology*. 1996; 70(2): 336-348.
28. Friedman J. Depression and posttraumatic stress response as outcomes of AIDS-related loss in gay male caregivers. PhD diss., Pacific Graduate School, 1998.
29. Shuchter SR, Zisook S. The course of normal grief. In Stroebe MS, Stroebe W, Hansson RO, eds. *Handbook of Bereavement: Theory, Research, and Intervention*. Cambridge: Cambridge University Press, 1993.
30. Bowlby J. *Loss: Sadness and Depression*. Vol. 3. London: Hogarth Press, 1980.
31. Worden JW. *Grief Counseling and Grief Psychotherapy: A Handbook for the Mental Health Practitioner*. New York: Springer Publishing Co., 1982.
32. Horowitz MJ. *Stress Response Syndromes*. 2d edition. Northvale, N.J.: Jason Aronson, 1986.
33. Lazarus RS, Folkman, S. *Stress, Appraisal, and Coping*. New York: Springer Publishing Co., 1984.
34. Holroyd KA, Lazarus RS. Stress, coping, and somatic adaptation. In Goldberger L, Breznitz S, eds. *Handbook of Stress*. New York: The Free Press, 1982.
35. Chesney MA, Folkman S. Psychological impact of HIV disease and implications for intervention. *Psychiatric Clinics of North America*. 1994; 17(1): 163-182.
36. American Psychiatric Association. *Diagnostic and Statistical Manual of Mental Disorders*. 4th edition. Washington, D.C.: American Psychiatric Association, 1994.
37. Rando TA. *Treatment of Complicated Mourning*. Champaign, Ill.: Research Press, 1993.
38. Raphael B. *The Anatomy of Bereavement*. New York: Basic Books, 1983.
39. Summers J, Zisook S, Atkinson JH, et al. Morbidity associated with Acquired Immune Deficiency Syndrome-related grief resolution. *Journal of Nervous and Mental Disease*. 1995; 183(6): 384-389.
40. Prigerson HG, Maciejewski PK, Reynolds CF, et al. Inventory of complicated grief: A scale to measure maladaptive symptoms of loss. *Psychiatric Research*. 1995; 59(1-2): 65-79.
41. Horowitz MJ, Bonanno A, Holen A. Pathological grief: Diagnosis and explanation. *Psychosomatic Medicine*. 1993; 55(3): 260-273.
42. Sikkema KJ, Koob JJ, Heckman TG. Prevalence and predictors of AIDS-related bereavement among HIV-infected men and women. Presentation from the Eighteenth Annual Meeting of the Society of Behavioral Medicine, San Francisco, 1997.
43. Erickson SE. Social support as mediator of emotional well-being in gay male caregivers of loved ones with AIDS. *Dissertation Abstracts International*. 1993; 55(7B): 3011.

44. Jacobs S, Grim K. Psychiatric complications of bereavement. *Psychiatric Annals.* 1990; 20(6): 314-317.
45. Martin JL, Dean L. Effects of AIDS-related bereavement and HIV-related illness on psychological distress among gay men: A 7-year longitudinal study, 1985-1991. *Journal of Consulting and Clinical Psychology.* 1993; 61(1): 94-103.
46. Schulz R, Visintainer P, Williamson G. Psychiatric and physical morbidity effects of caregiving. *Journal of Gerontology: Psychological Sciences.* 1990; 45(5): 181-191.
47. Mullan JT. The bereaved caregiver: A prospective study of changes in well-being. *The Gerontologist.* 1992; 32(5): 673-683.
48. Stylianos SK, Vachon MLS. The role of social support in bereavment. In Stroebe MS, Stroebe W, Hansson RO, eds. *Handbook of Bereavement: Theory, Research, and Intervention.* Cambridge: Cambridge University Press, 1993.
49. Maddison D, Walker WL. Factors affecting the outcome of conjugal bereavement. *British Journal of Psychiatry.* 1967; 113(503): 1057-1067.
50. Maddison D, Viola A, Walker WL. Further studies in conjugal bereavement. *Australian and New Zealand Journal of Psychiatry.* 1969; 3: 63-66.
51. Vachon MLS, Sheldon AR, Lancee WJ, et al. Correlates of enduring distress patterns following bereavement: Social network, life situation and personality. *Psychological Medicine.* 1982; 12(4): 783-788.
52. Mor V, McHorney C, Sherwood S. Secondary morbidity among the recently bereaved. *American Journal of Psychiatry.* 1986; 143(2): 158-163.
53. Vachon MLS. Identity change over the first two years of bereavement: Social relationships and social support in bereavement. PhD diss., York University, 1979.
54. O'Brien K. Primary relationships. Unpublished manuscript, Department of Psychology, Portland State University, 1992.
55. Nolen-Hoeksema S, Parker L, Larson J. The blessings and burdens of social ties: Social support and well-being in family members of the terminally ill. Unpublished manuscript, Department of Psychology, Stanford University, 1992.
56. Harvey CD, Bahr HM. Widowhood, morale, and affiliation. *Journal of Marriage and the Family.* 1974; 36(1): 97-106.
57. Sheldon AR, Cochrane J, Vachon MLS, et al. A psychosocial analysis of risk of psychological impairment following bereavement. *Journal of Nervous and Mental Disease.* 1974; 169: 253-255.
58. Atchley RC. Dimensions of widowhood in later life. *The Gerontologist.* 1975; 15(2): 1976-1978.
59. Martin JL, Dean L. Risk factors for AIDS-related bereavement in a cohort of homosexual men in New York City. In Cooper B, Helagson T, eds. *Epidemiology and the Prevention of Mental Disorders.* London: Routledge Press, 1989.
60. Neugebauer R, Rabkin JG, Williams JB, et al. Bereavement reactions among homosexual men experiencing multiple losses in the AIDS epidemic. *American Journal of Psychiatry.* 1992; 149(10): 1374-1379.
61 Silverman PR, Worden JW. Children's reactions to the death of a parent. In Stroebe MS, Stroebe W, Hansson RO, eds. *Handbook of Bereavement: Theory, Research, and Intervention.* Cambridge: Cambridge University Press, 1993.
62. Elizur E, Kaffman M. Factors influencing the severity of childhood bereavement reactions. *American Journal of Orthopsychiatry.* 1983; 53(4): 668-676.
63. Bass DM, Bowman K, Noelker LS. The influence of caregiving and bereavement support on adjusting to an older relative's death. *The Gerontologist.* 1991; 31(1): 32-42.

64. Norris FH, Murrell SA. Other adult family stress and adaptation before and after bereavement. *Journal of Gerontology*. 1987; 42(6): 606-612.

65. Rubin S. The resolution of bereavement: A clinical focus on the relationship to the deceased. *Psychotherapy*. 1985; 22(2): 231-235.

66. Weiss RS, Richards TA. A scale for predicting quality of recovery following the death of a partner. *Journal of Personality and Social Psychology*. 1997; 73(4): 851-854.

67. Folkman S, Lazarus RS, Gruen R, et al. Appraisal, coping, health status, and psychological symptoms. *Journal of Personality and Social Psychology*. 1986; 50(3): 571-579.

68. Carver CS, Pozo C, Harris SD, et al. How coping mediates the effect of optimism on distress: A study of women with early stage breast cancer. *Journal of Personality and Social Psychology*. 1993; 65(2): 375-390.

69. Coyne J, Aldwin C, Lazarus RS. Depression and coping in stressful episodes. *Journal of Abnormal Psychology*. 1981; 90(5): 434-447.

70. Folkman S, Lazarus RS. Stress processes and depressive symptomology. *Journal of Abnormal Psychology*. 1986; 95(2): 107-113.

71. Folkman S, Chesney M, Pollack L. Stress, control, coping, and depressive mood in human immunodeficiency virus-positive and negative gay men in San Francisco. *Journal of Nervous and Mental Disease*. 1993; 181(7): 409-416.

72. Stein N, Folkman S, Trabasco T, et al. Appraisal and goal processes as predictors of psychosocial well-being in bereaved caregivers. *Journal of Personality and Social Psychology*. 1997; 72(4): 872-884

73. Smith TW, Greenberg J. Depression and self-focus attention. *Motivation and Emotion*. 1981; 5(4): 323-331.

74. Smith TW, Ingram RE, Roth LD. Self focused attention and depression: Self evaluation, affect, and life stress. *Motivation and Emotion*. 1985; 9(4): 381-389.

75. Psyszcynski T, Holt K, Greenberg J. Depression, self focused attention, and expectancies for positive and negative future life events for self and others. *Journal of Personality and Social Psychology*. 1987; 52(5): 994-1001.

76. Nolen-Hoeksema S, Parker L, Larson J. Ruminative coping with depressed mood following loss. *Journal of Personality and Social Psychology*. 1994; 67(1): 92-104.

77. Nolen-Hoeksema S, McBride A, Larson J. Rumination and psychological distress among bereaved partners. *Journal of Personality and Social Psychology*. 1997; 72(4): 855-862.

78. Herek GM. Psychological heterosexism in the United States. In D'Augelli AR, Patterson CJ, eds. *Lesbian, Gay, and Bisexual Identities Over the Life Span*. New York: Oxford University Press, 1995.

79. Wagner G, Brondolo E, Rabkin J. Internalized homophobia in a sample of HIV-positive men, and its relationship to psychological distress, coping, and illness progression. *Journal of Homosexuality*. 1996; 32(2): 91-106.

80. Bandura A. *A Social Foundation of Thought and Action*. Upper Saddle River, N.J.: Prentice Hall, 1986.

81. Peterson C, Seligman MEP. Causal explanations as a risk factor for depression: Theory and evidence. *Psychological Review*. 1984; 91(3): 347-374.

82. Osterveis M, Solomon F, Green M, eds. Bereavement: Reactions, Consequences, and Care. Washington, D.C.: National Academy Press, 1984.

83. Jacobs S, Ostfeld A. An epidemiological review of the mortality of bereavement. *Psychosomatic Medicine*. 1977; 39(5): 344-357.

84. Wortman CB, Silver RC. Successful mastery of bereavement and widowhood: A life-

course perspective. In Baltes PB, Baltes MM, eds. *Successful Aging: Perspectives from the Behavioral Sciences.* Cambridge: Cambridge University Press, 1990.
85. McCrae RR, Costa PT. Psychological resilience among widowed men and women: A ten year follow-up of a national sample. In Stroebe MS, Stroebe W, Hansson RO, eds. *Handbook of Bereavement: Theory, Research, and Intervention.* Cambridge: Cambridge University Press, 1993.
86. Shuchter SR, Zisook S. Hovering over the bereaved. *Psychiatric Annals.* 1990; 20(6): 327-333.
87. Ruskin C. *The Quilt: Stories From the NAMES Project.* New York: Pocket Books, 1988.
88. Brown J, ed. *A Promise to Remember: The NAMES Project Book of Letters.* New York: Avon Books, 1992.
89. DuBois-Gadson R. Sharing the journey. *On Display: Newsletter of the NAMES Project Foundation.* 1998; 11(2): 19.
90. Burnell G, Burnell A. *Clinical Management of Bereavement: A Handbook for Healthcare Professionals.* New York: Human Sciences Press, 1989.
91. Shuchter S, Zisook S. Grief and mourning. In Jacobson J. *Psychiatric Secrets.* Philadelphia: Hanley & Belfus, 1996.
92. Lieberman M. Bereavement and self-help groups. In Stroebe MS, Stroebe W, Hansson RO, eds. *Handbook of Bereavement: Theory, Research, and Intervention.* Cambridge: Cambridge University Press, 1993.
93. Klein SJ. *Heavenly Hurts: Surviving AIDS-Related Deaths and Losses.* Amityville, N.Y.: Baywood Publishing Co., Inc., 1998.
94. Chesney MA, Folkman S. Psychological impact of HIV disease and implications for intervention. *Psychiatric Clinics of North America.* 1994; 17(1): 163-182.
94. Rando TA. Creating therapeutic rituals in the psychotherapy of the bereaved. *Psychotherapy.* 1985; 22(2): 236-240.
95. Sikkema KJ, Kalichman SC, Kelly JJ, et al. Group intervention to improve coping with AIDS-related bereavement: Model development and an illustrative case example. *AIDS Care.* 1995; 7(4): 463-475.
96. Elliott K. Introduction. The Hazelden Foundation. *The Twelve Steps of Alcoholics Anonymous.* New York: Hazelden Information Education, 1996.
97. Raphael B, Middleton W, Martinek N, et al. Counseling and therapy of the bereaved. In Stroebe MS, Stroebe W, Hansson RO, eds. *Handbook of Bereavement: Theory, Research, and Intervention.* Cambridge: Cambridge University Press, 1993.
98. Rando TA. Creating therapeutic rituals in the psychotherapy of the bereaved. *Psychotherapy.* 1985; 22(2): 236-240.
99. Horowitz MJ, Wilner N, Marmar C, et al. Pathological grief and the activation of latent self-images. *American Journal of Psychiatry.* 1980; 137(10): 1157-1162.
100. Eells TD. Relational therapy for grief disorders. In Barber JP, Crits-Christoph P, eds. *Dynamic Therapies for Psychiatric Disorders.* New York: Basic Books, 1995.
101. Barton D. The process of grief. In Barton D, ed. *Dying and Death.* Baltimore: Williams and Wilkins, 1977.
102. Zisook S, Shuchter S, Mulvehill M. Alcohol, cigarette, and medication use during the first year of widowhood. *Psychiatric Annals.* 1990; 20(6): 318-326.
103. Shuchter S, personal communication, 1999.

Index